MORE PRAISE FOR *RISK TO BLOSSOM*

"Reading this story of healing will certainly guide you toward your own. Take heart, you are entering a world of hope and transformation."
—Kimberly Lowelle Saward, Ph.D., president of The Labyrinth Society, and author of *Ariadne's Thread*

"Alice's writing touches gently on all aspects of life. She shows that any crisis is just part of your path to the center of your soul. Her journey from darkness to light proves that all the darkness in the universe can't diminish the light of a single candle."
—Rachelly Roggel, labyrinth artist and a contributor to *Invading Spaces: sexual violence against women*, Israel

"Thank you for your incredible work with what life offered you. Truly this is an inspiring story, and I am glad you are going to gift us with it."
—Christina Baldwin, author of *Calling the Circle*

& WHAT OTHER WOMEN SAY:

"Having shared the initiation with you, I carry a feeling of gratitude and a renewed sense of courage."
—Ali B., London, England

"The book is beautifully written...and was at times painful to read. There are points at which one just wants to reach out and cradle the writer, so strong is the pull."
—Claudia M., New York, N.Y.

"Thank you for all the work you do to help victims of sexual assault."
—Kerry N., Washington, D.C.

"*Risk to Blossom* will surely bring others the ability to move on to something much better in their lives; to realize that they are stronger than the brute event."
—Emma H., Tucson, Arizona

"What a wonderful book. It will change the lives of those who read it."
—Julie N., San Francisco, California

RISK TO BLOSSOM

[a journey of healing]

Alice Whytefeather

BLUE
CIRCLE
PRESS

San Francisco London

Blue Circle Press
P.O. Box 460055
San Francisco, CA 94146 USA

Library of Congress Cataloging-in-Publication Data

Whytefeather, Alice
Risk to blossom : (a journey of healing) / Alice
Whytefeather. -- 1st ed.
p. cm.
Includes bibliographical references.
ISBN 0-9669193-3-5
1. Whytefeather, Alice. 2. Rape victims--United
States--Biography. 3. Rape victims--Rehabilitation--
United States--Case studies. 4. Healing. 5. Labyrinths--
Religious aspects. 6. Meditations. 7. Authorship--
Psychological aspects. 8. Rape--United States--Case
studies. 9. Spiritual life. I. Title.
HV6561.W49 2004
364.1'532'092   2003116050

First Edition 2004

Printed in the United States of America
on acid-free paper

Book Design by Scribeworks

special thanks to Jasmin Cori
& Katherine Hernandez

for the silent ones
that they may be heard and healed

...& for the Angels,
with gratitude.

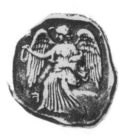

CONTENTS

Illustrations

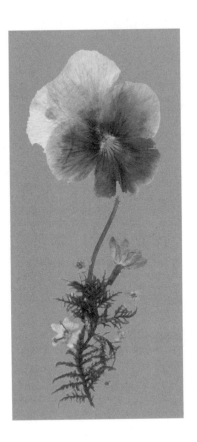

*Then the day came when the risk to remain tight in a bud
was more painful than the risk to blossom.*

ANAIS NIN

ꝑreface

This book is not about rape as a crime, but rather rape as an initiation. While to some this may seem a strange approach, to those of us who have had no choice, these words will be, at turns, provocative and familiar. Passing from an underworld of despair toward a place of greater self-knowledge, compassion, and awareness is not easy. Yet it is possible.

A true initiation brings with it unimaginable challenges. It is meant to shift consciousness, to inflict unwanted changes. Rape, for all its weighted sexual connotations, is in essence a violent, soul-shattering experience. This is especially true, as it was for me, if one's life is also threatened.

On my journey toward healing, there was much to learn and remember, as I reclaimed the lost parts of myself. I mourned the girl left behind, the maiden whose very survival sacrificed her innocence. By telling her story, I was finally able to acquaint myself with the woman—a bewildering alchemy—whom I have become.

This did not happen all at once. It took years. And I was often on this journey unawares. With few resting points and no sure place at which to arrive, it was (and is) an ongoing process of reconciliation. I have come to believe that for the survivor of any trauma, no matter how devastating and haunting the incident itself, a disguised blessing waits to be discovered.

Risk To Blossom was first written in London during the winter/spring of the year 2000, and then, after the words had settled a bit, completed in 2002. It was born of solitude, though often the words appeared unbidden, in unexpected flurries, while I walked through parks or rode the Tube. Other times, while lying in bed (either just as I drifted to sleep or during the first synapses of thought as I awoke), a few crucial sentences would dance across my mind, and I'd search the darkened flat for paper and pen. Many such scrawled notes, once deciphered, found their way to these pages. I regret that by using this spontaneous approach, I neglected to date entries; dates would have been helpful, providing anchors in a sea of words. Feeling an urgency similar to Scheherazade's, I have honored the power of intuition and present to you instead a chronicle of heart, mind, and spirit.

To say that this process has been one of discovery would be an understatement. It has been much more than that. I never intended to write such a book, nor did I really want to make such private information public. But truth is vain: It adores its own reflection and tricks its bearer into making such revelations as these by providing little mercies along the way.

During the writing, I began to feel a clearing within myself. If I had known that by risking the pain that comes with telling any traumatic story, I would inadvertently gain a sense of peace, I would not have waited for so many years. These words represent moments of grace as much as they do my stumbles along the path of consciousness. I hope they inspire you to confront your own shadows.

Part I

*Only those who know the knife
can understand the wound.*

MIRABAI

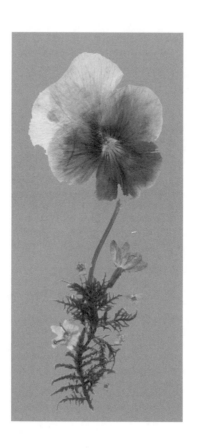

Sister of Religion

Not last night, but the night before,
twenty-four robbers came knocking at my door.
I asked them what they wanted, this is what they said:
Spanish Dancer, do the splits! The kicks!
Turn around, touch the ground—get out of town....

Childhood jump rope song

Children leave behind them a secret world, understood by them alone, and, as the years pass, often forgotten about. I do not know when I first heard about Peter Pan's Hideout, a mythic place in my neighborhood, nor exactly how I came to discover it. One day, when I was about six years old, I was drawn to a rocky trail off the side of the road, down past the oaks and lemon grass, to a shaded clearing. There I stood, motionless, surrounded by foliage—was it seconds, minutes, hours? A palpable benevolence twinkled through every leaf and infused the earth with fairy light. Everything shimmered with unworldly colors. I did not question it, feeling instead simultaneously tranquil and

7

amazed. I remember acknowledging to myself that something unordinary was occurring, though I had no reference point for the miraculous. Later, I felt perplexed when I brought my mother to what I thought was the same spot—there were the trees, the clearing—but the sense of enchantment was gone.

I was not a risk-taking child. Timid and introspective, I was given instead to philosophical daydreams. I was like Ferdinand the Bull, the storybook character who shied away from fighting, wanting only to smell the flowers. This meant that while other children were swinging jerkily from monkey bars or playing dodge ball, I was quietly off by myself wondering. I wanted to know not *why* we were here, but rather how deep the experience of life really went. Prompted by this curiosity, I once found myself running through a vast, golden field. My dainty expedition became more and more compelling as the familiar receded and all that was unknown and mysterious advanced. In the distance I could hear my father's concerned voice calling my name. I chose to ignore it. Because I sensed that just up ahead, on the other side of the field, past the fence...well, who knows what I thought was there, but there was an air of promise about it.

During dreams of flying, I would soar above our pink stucco house, dipping low then rising, yet always bound to the earth by an invisible force. On one occasion, I stood in the hall outside my bedroom. It was late at night; my parents were sleeping. The wooden gate meant to protect me from falling down the stairs was locked. I gently opened it. Was I dreaming? It didn't seem so. I surveyed the darkness for a while, gathering strength. Then

I levitated like a windblown feather, hovering over each step as I floated down. I remember my feet skimming the floor when I landed. Flying was a wondrous act, similar to leaving the body.

While Peter Pan's Hideout remained elusive, I did discover how to create my own sacred space under the swaying eucalyptus trees in my backyard. Typical of childhood play, this happened without much forethought or any sense of expectation. First I took a broom and swept the hardened California earth, so that its smooth undulations showed. Then I arranged a number of carefully selected stones in a circle. I placed myself in the center, where I sat alert and content. Something in me seemed to know about ritual, the sacredness of certain objects, and the healing magic of silence.

I was also drawn to the heady spectacle of the May Pole Dance, which was performed each spring by the girls of my elementary school. It took place on a grassy stage in a grove near an old, splintery stagecoach, a relic from the Gold Rush. Holding court in their tilted crowns were the May Day King and Queen, usually an unlikely pair forced together for the occasion. Parents watched us in our white blouses and pastel pinafores skip gaily around the pole and in between each other, weaving in and out as we followed the rings of chalk. If we did it right, the ribbons braided together in a colorful pattern. It was a pleasant, if complicated, dance during which I felt my sprouting self in all its glory. And then, having accomplished our task, we released the ribbons, reversed direction, and skipped back out again.

Of course, I didn't realize that this dance was

associated with the ancient springtime celebrations of many cultures. Creating a circle of stones and performing the May Pole Dance were just natural activities of childhood. Nevertheless, they planted within me a seed of awareness, which, however small, promised a later blossoming.

My spiritual roots are in Christianity. One of my earliest mystical experiences occurred when, as a girl, I glimpsed the sparkling blue gems of my cross necklace. More than an appreciation of the way the light caught the facets or the potent simplicity of the cross's form, it seemed

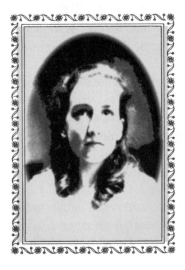

instead to trigger a recognition of the divine. A photograph taken at the time of my first communion shows me with a dutiful expression, gazing heavenward. Still, there must be something of the pagan in me too, for I have never required any more proof of God than a single flower.

I learned to pray in a charmed white chapel under the instruction of Reverend McConnell, who was the children's pastor. Standing before us in his long, black robe, he was the epitome of goodness. His melodic voice resonated with supreme and uncommon kindness, though I recall not one word of what he said. He seemed to love us. But what could he have been preaching to us about? We in his flock were all so small, unruly, and bewildered.

In kindergarten the line between the sacred and the profane came into brief focus then blurred when I received a kiss from the librarian's son. Inspired, I came home and sat scribe-like at the dining room table, recording on lined newsprint what was to be my first journalistic effort. Oddly, I felt as though I were not the child who had just experienced this clumsy sign of affection, but instead, the grown-up who, looking back from some future realm, recognized it as a turning point.

I guess I've always been a writer. From my earliest scribbles, I sensed the power of words, the importance of linking seen and unseen worlds. Writing was as engaging to me as listening to the braided sounds of a stream's rushing water. Although I was shy and rarely raised my hand in school, it seemed I had much to tell.

In the third grade, I wrote a report on the Pueblo Indians. I felt a curious connection to them. Why, for instance, did the act of grinding corn seem so familiar? It's true that I had heard stories about how the Indians had trusted Grandpa, inviting him to their sweat lodges. And there was a picture of a chief mixed with our family photos, along with some tiny, beaded moccasins. I used to visit Grandpa's ranch in Montana in the summers so may have been exposed to Indian life there (though by then they lived on reservations), but it seemed to go deeper than that. My report, titled "Religion of the Early Pueblos," was written with the innocence and clarity that only an eight-year-old can muster.

The early Pueblos believed that all live or dead objects had spirits. They also believed that the spirits would bring rain, luck at crops, no luck at crops, sickness or health, and they thought that they brought plain bad and good luck. When they smoked, they thought it would bring rain clouds. Prayer sticks are something the Pueblo Indians thought would bring rain too. The prayer stick is a piece of wood with a feather on top. The Indians put the prayer stick around farms and other places that need water. They also believed that feathers have a close relation to the sky, where the rain comes from. The Eagle flies among the clouds. The Eagle Dance is done in hopes the clouds will gather and it will rain. Snakes resemble lightning—so the Indians dance with snakes in their mouths. They say it brings rain. They think the snake carries their pleas to the Rain God. Singing is part of the Pueblo's religion. Their singing is part of ceremonies where they are dancing and praying for rain. Today some Indians are Christians, but all of them respect the ways of their ancestors.

By sixth grade, I was penning tales about death and the afterlife, signing them with the pseudonym Violet. The teacher who read them commented that their language was evocative of the sort of experiences one had while on acid (how did she know, I wonder?) Just as I was evolving as a writer, so was my interest in other realms steadily

12

growing.

When Maharishi Mahesh Yogi visited Squaw Valley, California in the 1960s, I was still a girl. I was there on a holiday with my parents. A group of people—devotees—had gathered, and we stopped to see what all the commotion was about. To our surprise, we saw a tiny brown man making his way toward us. Something made me step forward from the crowd and ask him for his autograph. He stopped and looked at me with the intensity of flame. Then he took the pencil and scrawled something in Hindi on the back of a paper napkin.

Because my parents were open-minded, I was allowed to attend Maharishi's talk that afternoon. I remember sitting on the floor along with the offerings of fruit and flowers. He spoke in a singsong voice about bliss, smiling constantly. I had the sense that he might rise up and float away.

Later, I became a Junior Deaconess. No longer attending lighthearted services in the children's chapel, I was now among the adults. The sermons were longer, more potent, yet all they caused in me was a drowsy sense of culpability and burden. I paraded before the congregation in a somber, theatrical manner. Accompanied by thundering organ music, I set the altar for Eucharist with holy bread and a silver chalice full of wine.

My spiritual development made a curious pit stop when, at my mother's prompting, I reluctantly joined Rainbow Girls, an organization related to the Freemasons. It was there that I was named the Sister of Religion. What this really meant was that I had certain lines to say at certain times during the meetings, and I was obliged to wear an orange sash. I don't remember much else, except that it was an uninspired time during which I tried to fit in, but failed.

During the 1970s, Sunday School evolved into an encounter group. We shouted out our teenaged frustrations, hit beanbag pillows, and then mirrored Christ by washing each other's feet. I first smoked marijuana on a church outing's overnight visit to the beach, floating over the dunes, laughing in darkness, as I dodged (or tried to) the molten wax of sand candles.

When I wasn't babysitting for a neighborhood commune or cutting class on rainy days so that I could write poetry, I was sequestered in my parent's basement, reading controversial books like *The Female Eunuch* and *Sisterhood is Powerful*. It was a passionate awakening. Seeing feminism as a religion in its own right, I created a manifesto about its virtues for my psychology class. Armed with pastel index cards which documented the various ways our lives were limited because of our gender, I debated the subject, defeating two backwards-thinking cheerleaders.

Around that time, followers of Maharishi Mahesh Yogi visited my high school, introducing us to Transcendental Meditation. I was impressed to learn that those who studied TM were each given a personal mantra. I spent some time pondering what mine might be, but came up with nothing.

Secret places, ancient rituals, and mumbled prayers all nourished the bud of my spiritual beginnings. And so I grew—curious, alone, quietly touched by the muse of writing, and awakened by the occasional glimmers of magic

I saw in the world.

Desire—whether for a person, knowledge, or an intangible *something*—can lead one to some very strange places. One can be on a quest, but not actually know it. I was well-embarked upon my own humble quest when, as a young woman, I decided to travel to Hawaii. Although this decision seemed small and inconsequential at the time, it significantly altered all that was to follow.

At the tender age of twenty, I learned that life has extraordinary depth. Unfortunately, this was associated with loss and evil, a fall from grace. That I survived such an experience has left me with the mark of gratitude, which, if I do not lose myself in the mundaneness of life, often serves me well, inspiring me to follow my heart and to always look deeper. Still, I would have preferred a happier instruction. Perhaps that child who once ran from her father is somewhere within me, innocently tracking mysteries.

The Path

On April 9, 1976, I was raped. There, I've said it.

Yet my story begins before then, and it continues into the present hour. It finds me kneeling before Volume II of the Oxford English Dictionary, magnifying glass in hand, seeking an impartial definition of that word.

> 1. *the act of taking anything by force;*
>   *violent seizure (of goods), robbery.*
> 2. *the act of carrying away a person,*
>   *especially a woman, by force.*
> 3. *violation or ravishing of a woman.*

Yes, true, I think, though *ravishing* conjures the helpless damsel of old-time movies who shrilly screams, faints perhaps. There must be another definition which takes into account the acted-upon, a way that describes the precarious rope-bridge one travels between a life-threatening experience and its aftermath. For survival is instinctive, automatic. It is the witnessing of one's potential death that summons the deepest fear, a fear that lingers by necessity, as though it were an amulet to ward off future danger.

Uncertain how to access this memory which has been my companion now for nearly twenty-five years, I close the dictionary, follow the path to the top of Primrose Hill, and study the shape-shifting clouds. It is a winter day in London. In the distance, the wheel of the London Eye slowly turns; behind me, a gathering of bare-leaved trees stands in shadows.

I have traveled thousands of miles to a place that couldn't be farther in spirit from Hawaii. There are no palm trees here, no macadamia nuts or ukuleles. Even in this land where I am once again a tourist, I feel a sense of home.

For all its crumbling, sooty history and its loveliness, London is, for me, a strangely maternal place. It comforts. In a cosmopolitan display of *feng shui* at its most quirky, church spires mingle with homely modern architecture and the Constable sky arches triumphantly over the hollow-pawed lions of Trafalgar Square. Nothing—not the bombs of World War II, the infiltration of The Gap and Starbucks, or the mobile phones wielded by the self-important as though they were dueling swords—can diminish this ancient city's good heart or its glory. Yet even as the kings and poets of past ages, now ghosts, pace Westminster Abbey, the blood lines of artist and aristocracy alike are imperceptibly thinning. There is a poignancy to the breathless pause between Big Ben's famous melody and the tolling of the hours, and the Thames's dark current can seem alternately wicked and sublime, as though its waters were the source of all dreams and passions. The city is changing. Politicians talk of pound and pence being replaced by the homogenous Euro.

London is an island, too, but other than this topographic similarity, it is nothing, nothing at all, like Hawaii. Maybe that is why I have come here to write: for the safety of its difference, for its neutrality.

I felt tempted by Hawaii, lured almost. There are reasons why a place speaks to one in such a manner, offering subtle warning. If we could learn to heed and obey such messages, our lives might take a different course.

Floater

Who was she? Twenty, waiflike, with sad blue eyes and long brown hair like that of a mermaid. My chief interest at that time was the drama of falling in and out of love. I wrote poetry, inspired by Sylvia Plath, Anaïs Nin, the Dadaists. I had no goals. My job in a San Francisco department store as a "floater" required me to fill in for the regular staff when they were ill or on vacation. I sold children's shoes, chocolate turtles, tennis rackets, whatever was needed. I was just beginning to realize that life, which fanned out miraculously before me, was much bigger than I was.

My uneasy blossoming (for I was often possessed by a profound shyness) was soon to be arrested by fate. Duplicitous fate has a way of appearing in the guise of ordinary events and circumstances, giving it more power in shaping the future than we may be aware of initially. A bus strike that spring made the commute downtown from my rented room on Potrero Hill difficult. Since I was already

19

chronically bored at my job waiting by the cash register, the prospect of not working was more of a relief than a disappointment. And with the offer of a free ticket (thanks to my father, who worked for an airline) tickling my sense of wanderlust, I had all the excuses I needed to visit my friend, Simon, in Hawaii.

I had first met Simon when I was still in high school in a small town in California. He was the cousin of a friend, older than I, a poet. He had developed his melancholia into an art. This was in the era of the Viet Nam war, and it occurs to me now that he might have been dodging the draft, for he was living in a cramped trailer the size of a cocoon in his aunt's backyard. One could sometimes hear the faint rain-like sound of his typewriter, evidence that he was in communion with his muse. Outside the trailer, peacocks marched across the weedy lawn, and dogs nuzzled and barked as young people gathered around Babu, the pet chimpanzee. There was also an iguana named Iggy. An aura of rural exoticism gave the house a welcome feeling, which always drew me to it.

Simon would periodically emerge, page in hand, eager to read what he had written. I was often the only willing audience. Many of his poems were about his estranged love, Iris, whom I imagined as a wise enchantress, with all the attributes of her namesake flower. The iris yawns open in spring to reveal its seductive petals, then, once pollinated, the petals shrivel and fall off. The same had happened, more or less, with Simon's Iris. At the very peak of his infatuation with her, she had turned cold and left him. Watching him mope about in his tie-dyed shirt and patched bell bottoms taught me much about the consequences of romantic love.

Simon explained how in Greek mythology Iris was known as the goddess of the rainbow. Looking much like an angel in her brightly colored robe and halo of light, she sped across the sky or descended to the underworld, the bearer of divine messages. I was more intrigued by the real Iris, for she had mired his poems with longing and had given his already sensitive eyes a look of urgency. It was hard not to be jealous of a woman so carelessly powerful.

Once, Simon and I walked in the nearby field, he in his great black hat, like fellow Irishman Oscar Wilde— perhaps he also wore a cape, held his hand over his heart. I was full of awe and curiosity. What did it mean to be a poet? We paused beside one of the trees that had been part of my childhood—a gnarled grey oak, the subject of nightmares—for one of those conversations about which nothing can later be remembered, except that a bond was formed. Perhaps he sympathized with my plight: I was yearning to escape the dominance of an overprotective mother. He, in turn, was drawn to Hawaii (where Iris was). We were both unsettled. Plans and possibilities filled the air.

Our encounter was followed-up by letters over a span of two years, the first of which was intended to reach me at my parent's home. It never did. Instead, a week before I moved out, I received an anonymous note.

A letter addressed to you was put in my box by mistake and almost destroyed by my 2 year old. I have salvaged the address of the person who wrote it and am

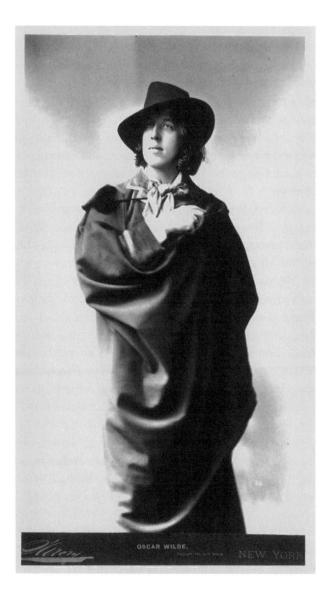

OSCAR WILDE.

NEW YORK

sending it to you.

An inauspicious beginning. But it proved that Simon had made it to paradise. A few months later, an airmail letter arrived at my new San Francisco address.

It's good that you're out now and on your own and with good people...I have felt you near me in recent weeks. You know that I miss you, don't you? The past year has offered me opportunities here, and now they are panning out...I'm like the sea in that I sometimes make waves to clear water...

Other letters, usually typed, though sometimes in his backhanded handwriting, followed.

I see it! You and me, and I feel as you did when we first met, and as I hope you do now...

I've thought it over and I think we can work it out, but first try to understand. Iris and I are splitting... The situation is tense...it will be getting heavy, so be ready for anything...

Then a poem, conjuring a vision of Persephone.

*...eyes, seeing you, amid the memory
spilling wild of flowers across the field...*

His last letter promised that, now Iris was gone, things would be different for us because his job was his only distraction. He also mentioned a "money interest" and how Hawaii was "a great place to party."

There is no absolute to anything. I believe that amid the crashing madness there is that moment of pause, to hold us in the light.

This was the existential Simon who had initially attracted me, who inspired me to glimpse life's rough yet beautiful edges. Despite my apparent conquest, I felt oddly detached, rather like a kitten who had caught a mouse but lacked the experience to know how next to behave. Still, I was curious.

I can make no promise as to great wealth, or a Rolls limo...it wouldn't be like before, we would be together this time...No surprises tho', I can do better without them, but I really do want you to come...you can only meet somebody so many times, before you realize that you are supposed to know them...

I don't need to say anymore—.
Love, Simon.

Don't Go

From the moment I stepped onto the plane and waved to my friends from the window of First Class, toasting them with my champagne-and-orange juice cocktail, I was aware of the whisper of a premonition, which seemed to say, *Don't go.*

I had grown up hearing stories about the sixth sense and divine intervention from my Romanian-American mother. Once, on an impulse, Grandpa had decided to quit his job at the mine in Montana. This was strange behavior for an immigrant who valued work and desperately needed it. After he had turned in his papers and walked down the road to no doubt wonder what he had done, the mine blew up, killing all of his fellow miners. Another time, during World War I, an explosion rocked the field where he stood, leaving him its only survivor. Grandpa also had prescient dreams. In one, a good friend appeared to him just before news came that he had unexpectedly died.

Don't go. The difficulty in heeding an intuition is that it is rarely, if ever, grounded in reason. Gradually my apprehension quieted. I began to enjoy the flight and looked forward to seeing Simon.

A Hurried Lullaby

I see myself carrying a small plaid suitcase. I was hopeful, though not overly so. Diamond Head, the island's dormant volcano, loomed before me. The sweet scent of coconut oil and overripe pineapples filled the balmy air.

Because Simon was working, I traveled by bus from the airport, past industrial-type buildings and fields of sugarcane, to the shabby suburbs where he lived. To my surprise, it was quite far from Waikiki Beach, where couples wearing fragrant leis strolled along the lantern-lit promenade to luaus of *poi* and roasted pig, smiling dreamily at the hula dancers. This was a different world entirely, full of broken-down cars, roving children, and plump women in muumuus.

I remember seeing a book about psychics at Simon's when I first arrived. I opened it to a photograph of Madame Blavatsky, the Russian occultist, hand resting on her cheek, shawl around her head, that formidable, all-knowing stare. Slowly I turned the pages, absorbing with a sudden thirst

27

all the images and information. When I raised my head, there was my host: thin and tanned, owlish is his wire-rimmed spectacles.

"Aloha!" he said with a smile. It is a blessing of love, a word that means both hello and goodbye in the Hawaiian language.

I blinked at my surroundings. Simon's apartment, though spacious, felt oddly stifling. Papers—poems, I supposed—wilted beside his typewriter. Maybe it was due to the humidity trapped in the shadowy rooms.

Later, he led me upstairs, showed me the bed. Not much else was in the room, which bore the lonely mark of a bachelor. There was a window to one side with thin orange curtains. A wicker chair. Also a small white bathroom and a closet near the top of the stairs. Somehow I already knew that we, as a couple, were probably not meant to be, but I still intended to play my part in the romantic drama. After dinner, we opened up and talked about ourselves. Maybe he, too, realized that there was no future for us. Or maybe not.

"I'm a good guide," he said. He mentioned hikes we could take, waterfalls we could visit. He must have said a hundred things, all of which are now obliterated by an avalanche of unwanted memory.

Soon we were lying together on his bed. The heat made us lazy. *In the wastelands of these sheets, mere hands lack labor and move about like friends*, I would later write in a poem. We kissed—soft, damp, vague, exploratory—an attempt to seal our tenuous relationship. Yet even in the depths of our sincere and burrowing hugs, I sensed the absence of something crucial. Chemistry? Passion? Or was it the presence of something unwanted—-the ghost of Iris?

The next day, around noon, we were on our way to visit one of Simon's favorite places. He wouldn't tell me anything more, preferring to keep me in suspense. I imagined possibilities. Would it be a romantic cliff-side perch, veiled in ferns, plumeria, and hibiscus? A dark cave filled with upside-down bats? Or maybe he would lead me along a precarious footpath to a beach of that virgin black sand I'd heard about. No matter where one went on the island, the shushing, aqua ocean was never far away. It crept up along the coral reefs and then retreated, sucking in its sudden breath. Undertows swept away swimmers, while eels slithered among starfish. And there was always the possibility of a *tsunami*, that great water dragon which could stand taller than any building. The ocean's restrained, unfathomable power encroached on one's being, eroding any presumed separation between it and you.

We had packed a lunch of fruit and potato chips. Simon had also brought along a canteen of water. What more did we need? The fickle morning showers had passed, leaving the air cleansed, yet full of pristine fragrances. As we walked, I anticipated the lazy hours ahead. Once we arrived at wherever we were going, there would be nothing for us to do but to relax, to peel back the pliant skin from mangoes, to enjoy the novelty of each other's company, and, if we felt like it, to plot our hazy future.

A tall, sandy-haired man stood in our path.

"Hullo—, " said Simon, bobbing to a stop.

I waited while the two of them talked. Simon's

hair, which was parted down the middle, hung about his somber face, Christ-like. I watched him tuck a lock of it behind one ear, then smooth a hand over the top of his head, as though to dispel the knot of energy that was forming between them.

We were at the border of Simon's neighborhood, near a stand where a few zombie-like tourists examined souvenirs. I thought of the nearby Royal Hawaiian Hotel with its pink bell towers and fairy-tale wrought iron gates, which I had seen once before on a trip with my parents. But this time was different. There was Simon—tender, attentive, doggedly sincere. Maybe it could be good between us. I would never go home. I would stay in Hawaii forever.

Traveling shifts one, too easily, between dimensions. Here I was witness to a different culture, with its mysterious Polynesian roots. I was a stranger, conspicuous in my floppy, blue-and-white checked sunhat, bikini under tee shirt, shorts, and towel sarong, and a pair of thongs on my pale feet. There is an ease that comes from the shedding of work clothes and nylon stockings, an unhindered feeling of sublime liberation. I would have been feeling that then.

The sun blazed overhead with a white heat. I squinted up at the silhouette of the towering man. Like a giraffe casually munching leaves, he had a way of deliberately leaning in toward Simon as he spoke from the side of his mouth. He was talking in a hushed monotone, which I could not hear.

"It wasn't me, man," Simon said coolly.

At some point, I must have been introduced as a

friend visiting from San Francisco, but apparently this fellow existed in a different stratosphere where such information was unimportant. He made no eye contact whatsoever—not even with Simon—which I found peculiar at the time and especially disturbing when, much later, I pulled apart the memory of our encounter, looking for clues.

And then he turned abruptly and walked away. If Simon felt intimidated by his strange acquaintance (whose reign in the island's underworld of drugs and prostitution was as yet unknown to me), he didn't show it. Instead, he gave my hand a squeeze, and we carried on. Taking his cue, I accepted the fact that Simon knew such an unpleasant person, just as I accepted his family's haphazard zoo of peacocks, iguana, and chimpanzee. Besides, the man I had just met had nothing to do with me. Or did he?

Although we had paused for only a moment, it was one of those seemingly innocent occurrences—like that misdirected letter nearly devoured by a two-year old—which changed everything. An alarm should have sounded, but didn't. Some inner warning system ought to have begun wildly beeping, but that didn't happen either—not yet, anyway.

All I really remember is glancing up at him in that obscure, yet oddly precise moment. Did I know then that he had recently been released from prison for breaking and entering into the theatre arts building where Simon worked? That he believed it was Simon who had turned him in? I must have learned all this later, from a mild and sheepish Simon, who was too late in protecting me.

"Gotta go!" he called. "Be back late, my love, around

2 a.m. See you in the morning." Simon was moonlighting as a taxi cab driver. As the door closed, I pictured him taking strangers between airport and hotels, making conversation, collecting tips. I was alone in the quiet of his apartment. I made a cup of peppermint tea and tried to type a few letters, but I felt at odds, unfocused. Writer's block? After tearing up my attempts, I decided to go to bed.

I changed into my sheer blue nightgown. Then I did a strange thing: I took the money and identification from my purse and hid them in my checked sunhat. I put a small amount of cash—about sixteen dollars—out in the open. My purse I left downstairs, bundled beneath a sweatshirt. There was no reason for this. It was just intuition, whispering its hazy warning.

I stood for a moment in the kitchen, still at odds. Then feeling an overwhelming urge to write a poem, I returned to the typewriter. I typed a title, *a hurried lullaby*, and words began to appear on the page in a gallop, as though summoned there by someone else. Certainly I had no idea what I was writing, or why.

> *a cord,*
> *a sailor's cord tying knots in a different way,*
> *an ugly bulge beneath sails of an indifferent nature.*
> *swoop of destiny in the air...*
>
> *take this sunset from my hands,*
> *it only turns them orange.*
> *let me diagnose this day's intentions:*

A Hurried Lullaby

the miracles that miscarried,
stolen goods,
a crushable tophat out of my reach,
the bloated life that leaks...

a quick fish gets the bait
moves in the sluggish sea
where mermaids pause in the gift of light.

curtains heave and change the air
i run downstairs.
guard this afternoon from night,
it makes the bathwater go cold
and lets the sun slide away.
too playful, too easy for the chains to rattle
and wake me.
turn away and take ten steps—

can you imagine a worse way to begin?

You Can't Always Get What You Want

I resist telling my story. Why invoke those ghosts? It feels unsafe. I want to protect the girl in her blue nightgown. And yet I know I can't.

I doubt that I said a prayer that night. Certainly not the prayer of my childhood—*Now I lay me down to sleep, / I pray the Lord my soul to keep. / If I should die before I wake, / I pray the Lord my soul to take.*—which had always seemed unnecessarily ominous, infusing bedtime with a spell of danger. No, after a last sip of tea and a click of the light, I was lulled to sleep by the moist, tropical heat, the swishing palm fronds. Drifting ever so gently into sweet, nocturnal oblivion...

When next I woke, two men were standing over my bed.

"Hello!" I said in a high voice. The room was dark, and in my confusion I assumed that they were Simon and someone else. I was wrong. Whoever they were, they appeared to be startled and jerked backwards, saying that

34

they thought *I* was Simon.

"We're friends of his," one ventured.

"He's at work," I said. "He won't be back until later."

"We'll wait."

They gave the impression of being drunk. More than once they apologized for intruding, laughing as they staggered in and out of the bathroom and the closet (mistaking it for the bathroom), finally coming to lean against the banister, opposite me.

"Why don't you wait downstairs?" I asked. I felt confused, annoyed, a shade apprehensive. Maybe this was a dream?

No, they wanted to talk. Politely. One was tall and angular, the other short and dark. For the purpose of this story, I will call them Hyena and Dark One. I didn't recognize the taller one as the same unfriendly man whom I had met with Simon.

There was a catfight outside, so they got up, came over by the bed and looked outside at the yard below. Wearily, just long enough to sigh, I glanced in the opposite direction. Then all at once, they turned. Hyena pulled out a long-bladed knife, and they both swooped near. I shrieked, and one of them hissed, "Shut up, or you'll get it!" They were sober now; their earlier inebriated behavior had only been an act, a deception.

Suddenly I was punched, hard, on the right side of my face. I saw a flurry of stars and disappeared into a pit of dizziness, crying out where no one could hear me.

There must have been a guardian angel with me that night, a benevolent entity with wings the color of flame and eyes so steady as to be unwavering. It would have sensed the manifestation of evil and appeared at my defense. When they asked, "Where's your money, your ID?" their voices sharp and sly, the angel would have stood between us, wings spread, denying them their power. While one held the knife at my neck and the other searched the room like a dog mesmerized by the scent of the hunt, the angel would have held a narrow finger to its lips. *Don't worry.*

But I was beyond that.

They found the sixteen dollars and some money of Simon's. "Where's your purse?"

"I don't know." My voice sounded far off.

"When Simon gets back, we want you to stay quiet."

Quiet... I inwardly repeated.

"Because we're going to kill him."

So the knife had been intended for him. Had I not woken precisely when I did, I would have been killed in my sleep.

A knife has no other purpose but to cut or stab. Unless perhaps as decoration. This knife was cold and hard. It moved quickly. Moments ago I had seen its supernatural glint as it parted the air around it.

Their anger rose and fell in waves. I glanced at the clock. Simon wouldn't be home for hours.

Hyena sat on the left side of the bed, while Dark One unzipped his trousers. Hawaiian music blared outside. The curtains swelled.

* * *

I have struggled to find the right words to describe what happened next, writing it one way, and then another. Nothing has seemed right—not the tangle of verbs, hanging like empty nets, or the well-meaning adjectives which seemed pitifully melodramatic. It is like trying to show someone the eye of a hurricane without benefit of swirling wind, without any real threat of danger or loss, but only the relative calm available in retrospect.

That night reality assumed a density that I have, thankfully, never encountered again. Present, past, and future merged to form one all-encompassing experience outside the normal boundaries of time, immeasurable by even the most brilliant physicist. For this alone, it was extraordinary, life-changing. A pocket of time opened, holding me within it. The telling of this experience creates a challenge for the writer in me. Memory has captured images that defy yet demand common description. How to salvage the appropriate blend of coherence and incoherence from the sound of him unzipping his trousers and the horror induced by that single, mundane act. One phrase keeps returning to me: *In the darkness, my body became blind.*

But blind to whom? Certainly I was seen by him— Dark One—as he tugged back the sheet and forced my sunburnt legs apart. I must have been not only seen, but felt. Maybe, for him, it was an erotic moment, though I doubt it. I suspect he was acting out of pure aggression, opportunism, frightened himself of what he was about to do—though not frightened enough to stop. What *I* felt was not purely physical or emotional, but rather something belonging to a different realm. Rape has its own vocabulary. It was new, unnatural, unwanted; I did not want to learn to speak it. This alone was cause for a profound dread which, in my semi-conscious state, I could not understand or interpret, but merely sensed, as one half-asleep might perceive a fire burning nearby—that first unmistakable twinge that something's amiss, a sense that can quickly escalate into hysteria.

Like a vulture stimulated by an ancient, ingrained violence, he descended upon me. I didn't scream or struggle. I didn't fight back. Instead, with each of his greedy, purposeful thrusts, a part of me retreated.

The knife's edge rested at my throat, a quivering compass needle pointing to danger. This was my life—fragile, sacred, crystalline—at the mercy of strangers. I held my breath, falling to a place deep within where air was not needed.

Shock is a great protector: It reduces to a single heartbeat that which is horrific and incomprehensible. It temporarily reduces the pain of such an assault upon body and spirit. As shock descended, I began to feel oddly numb and neutral. A ball of energy surrounded me, a hazy glow offering a mantle of protection. It was like a presence that was a link between worlds. I was simultaneously aware of it and of the billowing curtains behind me, rhythmically filling with air, releasing, the haunted, operatic sound of feral cats outside.

Then my perspective changed. I was hovering over the bed, watching events unfold with detached clarity. I could see the darkened window, the stairs, the tops of the men's heads. ("Tie her up," one of them was saying.) I could see the girl, splayed like a starfish, half-clad in her thin blue nightgown. She was shaking uncontrollably.

Now *I* was shaking with tremors of panic, lightning bolts of fear. A visceral, wordless knowledge informed me that there was no escape. Time had unmercifully stopped, like a jinxed clock that would never start again.

A door opened and closed. Simon was home. They warned me to keep quiet, and, like an acrobat performing a trick, Dark One neatly rolled off me and crouched on the floor. Hyena disappeared into the closet, while Simon slowly walked upstairs. There is nothing slower than the sound of a man walking toward his doom. When he reached the top of the stairs, he looked in my direction. I looked back, but across the unlit room we couldn't really see each other.

Out of the closet jumped Hyena. Dark One stayed nearby, holding me down.

Chaos. A blur of struggling figures, wild, incoherent shouts. If they killed Simon, they would probably do the same to me. They wouldn't want to leave a witness.

I must have looked away. Yet I could still hear Simon's voice, desperately pleading, trying to defend himself. Words snaked back and forth between them, around and around, knotting in conflict, stretching so taut they seemed sure to break. Simon must have somehow convinced them of his innocence—*It wasn't me, man*—because eventually they all went downstairs. For a moment, I thought I was safe. And then Hyena appeared. Alone. Was he still carrying his knife? I don't remember.

My glimpse of the thin membrane that separates

39

life from death lasted far longer than I would have wished. Hours passed. Reality shattered into fragments of uncertainty. In such circumstances, fear is a luxury. It was the *not knowing* how it would end that disturbed me. In all those hours, I had not one full thought, only a continuous, helplessly imploding realization of my mortality.

Dark One had returned. He was smaller in stature, but more muscular than Hyena. His skin glistened like wax. When his movements quickened during his orgasm and then abruptly stopped, I felt baffled by his intense expression. His eyes glassy, his taut face a demon's mask. It was as though he were looking through me. Yes, *through* me, to a place where I did not exist. I had disappeared. Or was I already dead?

By dawn, they had made a deal: Simon would give them the keys to his cab and meet them later in the week with guns. We would not call the police. There were other assorted promises. And then they were gone.

"I'm sorry," said Simon. "I'm so sorry..."

A faint light filled the room. There was a mark on the sheet, my panties were wet with semen, and there was a crushed cigarette butt on the floor.

I turned on a radio to find out what time it was. A song was playing by The Rolling Stones: *You can't always get what you want...*

Through the cathedral-like windows of this London flat, I watch a flock of birds swirl through rain clouds. How curiously small and insignificant they seem.

That was then, this is now, I remind myself,

40

gathering my wool cape around me. I am cold, my temples throb. I have a headache. Memory forms an irresistible bridge which is sometimes too painful to cross.

"There is but one light, and there is but one darkness," proclaims an old Siamese proverb. Yes, I think, and toward dawn sometimes, when one least expects it, light and darkness almost merge.

Scarab

We decided to leave Hawaii that morning. With a burst of retroactive paranoia, I locked the doors and closed the windows. Then I checked my sunhat and under the sweatshirt. I was lucky; except for the sixteen dollars, they hadn't found my money, ticket, or identification.

"But I don't have any cash," said Simon vaguely, as he gathered up some of his things.

"Never mind," I said. I was high on adrenaline. "I'll call some friends in California. We'll find a way."

We stepped outside. I peered up at the sky, felt the sun's warm embrace, then checked all around, afraid of being out in the open. We must have looked a pair: no sleep, my face bruised and swollen, Simon lugging his typewriter.

I called a number of people collect. "An emergency," I said before swiftly becoming mute. I just couldn't explain what had happened, though there must have been panic in my voice, when I repeatedly asked them to "please wire money."

"Huh? Sorry..." Either it was too early in the morning, everyone was broke, or perhaps, because of my lack of detail, they assumed I was having romantic difficulties—or crying wolf.

Finally my first love and friend, Henry, came on the phone. He was a student on food stamps with little to spare. "Sure," he said, in that calm voice of his. "I can help."

There was no real transition, no time to think or feel, between what had happened and our arrival in San Francisco. We walked out the door like refugees, carrying only a few belongings. I hadn't showered or eaten. Somehow I had the presence of mind to snap a photograph of the outside of the apartment.

I also noted, with a twisted sense of humor, the Snow White display in the Honolulu airport. She too was a victim of a plot to kill (by poison apple), but at least she had a Prince Charming to revive her from her death-sleep. It hardly seemed Simon qualified for that. His reaction, while effective in that it contributed to keeping us alive, was far from heroic. Nor were there any comical dwarfs— no Bashful, Grumpy, or Sneezy. And, with my still-tender cheek the marbled colors of the interior of an abalone shell, there was no question that I was *not* "the fairest of them all."

I remember ordering a pastry—a bear claw—in the airport coffee shop while we waited for Simon's ticket to come through, and the elderly couple who glanced at us blankly as we walked past their booth. I remember nothing about the flight.

* * *

With Simon in tow I returned to the same rented room on Potrero Hill. It was a time of feeling simultaneously angry to have been violated, yet grateful to be alive— though mostly I just felt nothing. I couldn't communicate to Vanessa, my high-spirited roommate, the depth of what had happened.

I had known Vanessa since eighth grade when she had appeared at my school in a tattered sailor dress. Resembling an albino with her white skin and unusual curly white hair, it would have been impossible *not* to notice her. But it was her great, gap-toothed smile and her ability to laugh at herself that made the idea of being her friend hard to resist. We lived two houses away from each other and each misty morning walked drowsily to the bus stop together.

Vanessa is of Italian descent. Her family tree, which is peopled with innumerable aunts, uncles, cousins, and step-relatives, is especially convoluted. She had once been a ward of the court, passed between families, finally settling with her father, red-headed step-mother, Asian step-brother, two great danes, and a Siamese cat called Ting-a-Ling.

Her room was rather like a nun's quarters, its only objects a small bed and a ceramic bowl. Vanessa cherished that bowl. She had bought it with money that she had earned, and it seemed to represent something to her— permanence, maybe.

Because we were teenagers, we laughed constantly, and often got into mischief. Once, while furtively drinking Cointreau in the school lavatory, we heard the alarm of a fire drill, stumbled out the door, turned in the wrong direction, and found ourselves in the path of two-thousand fleeing students.

These days her focus was on transforming our ramshackle house on Potrero Hill with its peeling linoleum and derelict front yard into a quaint Victorian, complete with wood stove and oriental carpets. The house was shared with her boyfriend, myself, a cat, and an easily-agitated German shepherd. And now Simon.

While Vanessa refinished chairs and decided on wallpaper, I hid in my attic bedroom, feeling claustrophobic whenever Simon ducked in to look at me mournfully. It was in that dark, olive-colored room where the cat decided to have her kittens, her small grey face timid and strained as she suckled them, and where I spent hours by the window, wishing for a different view.

Only one person had even a partial understanding of what I'd experienced, but Simon, uprooted and shaken himself, reminded me of what I could not speak of. I felt suffocated in his presence. Wasn't it his fault, anyway? Hadn't he invited me to Honolulu? So I asked him to go. I watched him scuffing toward the door like a scolded puppy. His face was ashen, his eyes downcast. He seemed thinner. I didn't ask him where he was going. I didn't care.

I needed more time and space around me. Although I didn't know it at the time, I also needed to heal. Yet it would take nearly twenty-five years and a journey of six-thousand miles for that process to truly begin.

The bruise on my face turned rainbow shades— from purple to green to a sickly amber—faded, and then disappeared. In the mirror I looked the same as before. I had the same boring, dead-end job, same friends. The same life.

While outside the world carried on as before, inside, my spirit had been startled awake. It had seen too much. So death was really only a breath, a heartbeat, away. And evil was a greater power than I had ever dared admit.

Not long after the incident in Hawaii, I decided to tell Simon's aunt what had happened. Strong and taciturn, she was married to a cranky man who, with his long beard, squinty eyes, and pipe, resembled a lumberjack (in fact, he would die of a heart attack while chopping a tree). It was in the family's backyard that Simon had lived in his teardrop trailer. Their troupe of fiercely physical children all hiked and camped. I had been an only child. Timid to a fault, possessing an inborn fear and reverence for the outdoors, I was in every way their opposite.

Returning to the town where I had grown up, I followed the familiar, rambling neighborhood road known as "the circle," which had connected my house with Vanessa's and our other friends. It was a mission of truth, a way to validate, and somehow purge myself of, the unbelievable. Planning my speech as I walked, I was led to the aunt's door, where I breezed in. It took all of five minutes to recount the information. "And then they raped me," I said. This was in a time when public confessions of such intimate details were not commonplace. It was before Oprah. When I finished, there was a strange silence between us. What did I expect from her? Nothing, really. I just knew that I had to tell. Still, her response mystified me.

She sat for a moment, recalling with a nervous laugh the time I had fallen from their backyard swing, hit my head, but hadn't cried. Then she calmly got up and went into the next room. I could hear her rummaging about. When she returned, she presented me with an Egyptian scarab. The scarab is an ancient amulet. It represents immortality and resurrection; the Egyptians considered it sacred. When someone died, they placed the scarab in their tomb as a symbol of new life. This was a black scarab on a dainty gold chain. I thanked her for it, then turned my attention to its small, beetle-like shape in my palm. It gave me a dark and empty feeling. Not only was it an unattractive necklace, but it seemed to signify a closure which I sensed was more for her benefit than for mine. She had reciprocated, yes—her cursed-looking antique for my confession—but there was no apparent feeling involved for either of us. Still, even this surreal formality was preferable to my mother's hysteria; *she,* I imagined, would have compounded the situation, making it worse than it already was. Perhaps, in lieu of love, the scarab's healing power would affect me without my knowledge. So I wore the necklace for a while. Then one day, just as curiously as it had come to me, it disappeared.

A friend's mother who also lived in the circle and had learned from Simon's aunt what had happened offered to take me to a counseling session. I cheerfully accepted. Yet by then, I had already masked the shock, even from myself. I was flippant, unfocused. Again I told my story, making little flourishes to emphasize the knife, its sudden power over me, but I felt nothing. No tears.

That I had survived was all that really mattered.

Although I had received just one counseling session myself, I at one point decided to become a rape crisis center volunteer. I was deflected from that calling by the generic terminology: *Rapist. Victim.* I didn't see myself as a victim, and I knew that those two, as evil as they had been that evening, were men, had once been boys, had dreams and fears, just like myself. Dangerous and misguided, yes, but the word "rapist" branded them, denying them their humanity, and in so doing, denied me mine. Even in my quiet rage, I knew that they were more than that.

Even worse, they had names. Simon had given them to me reluctantly, uncertain of their correctness. I look at these names now, scrawled in blue ink. After each name, there are notes, written by me: *out on bail, grand theft, breaking and entering.*

When I had called the San Francisco police, the switchboard operator had transferred me to a department called "Sex Detail." They, in turn, had instructed me to contact the police in Hawaii. That had seemed impossible; the distance between here and there was separated by thousands of miles of water. I had escaped, I didn't want to go back. I couldn't. That distance, and only that, protected me.

And so I forgot about Simon, the two men, and their criminal records. I forgot about that girl and her invisible wounds.

A few years passed. Then one afternoon, Simon appeared at my new apartment in San Francisco which I was sharing with Henry. He was polite, but he looked worried. I think he needed to prove to himself that I was still alive. Reaching into his pocket, he sheepishly said that he had written a poem for me about my April.

48

Scarab

There are times
When faith hath no healing,
Patience no time,
Caring no concern.
When touched by this illness,
Not seeing for the light,
I am only, barely
Comforted in my fright.
I have had my failures.
Somewhere still,
My wreath is kept.
I never know what
I've hoped for,
Nor dreamed when I
Have slept:
But always there is an urging,
And always I will try,
But somewhere in my weakness,
Small pieces of me die.

Flood

A writer's life is rumored to be a solitary one. Yet to me it is the reverse. Memories and dreams crowd out any loneliness. My mind is a storehouse of words. Stories present themselves to me, asking to be told. It is always a relief when the ego briefly forgets itself and one is suspended in "the zone."

But even this zone is often infiltrated by reality. Needing a break from my writing, I turn on the TV. The people who have survived the recent flood in Mozambique are clinging to rooftops and trees. Standing here, in this London flat, waiting for the tea kettle to boil, it is difficult to imagine their fear and horror and anguish. Somehow the greater the number of victims involved in such a catastrophe, the easier it is to distance oneself. The one blurs into the many. So I imagine *one* woman, the wet torn clothes against her skin, the cramp in her stomach, the slippery wood under her hand. Maybe she has a child and her husband is missing. Perhaps her greatest trauma—

beyond physical discomfort—is that she doesn't know how her story will end. She doesn't know if the water will continue to rise, whether she will survive. Or not.

I say a prayer for her, then change the channel. The peace process has broken down in Ireland, again. The weather is dull, with sunshine predicted tomorrow.

Scheherazade

The path toward healing appeared and disappeared from view in a synchronistic fashion. Sometimes I followed it; other times, I turned away. Often I made my life more difficult than it needed to be. Oblivious to the depth and complexity of my wound, I never consciously sought to heal myself. I didn't know that the rape was fermenting. I assumed that with the passage of time—six months or so—I would be mostly healed. It didn't happen like that.

California during the 1980s became the heart of the New Age movement. Friends, strangers, and teachers regularly came into my life with knowledge and information from which I benefited. I met astrologers, tarot card readers, palmists, psychics, shamans, est graduates, gurus, yoga masters, followers of the Fourth Way, Sufis, Rosicrucians, and Buddhists. I was also introduced to that oracle known as the *I Ching*, or *Book of Changes*, which has remained a cherished companion. All offered pieces to the puzzle of life, pieces which I arranged and rearranged in my own way. It wasn't so much that I was seeking something (perhaps it was seeking me); rather, I was enchanted by the widening mystery.

Belly dancing is a woman's dance. As erotic as it is graceful, it represents the act of childbirth. Dancing to the ancient music of the Middle East initiated me into the cult of the female. I joined an amateur dance troupe, sewed a costume of glittery coins and bright, flamboyant colors, and learned to play the finger cymbals. With each twirl and dip of the veil, I became myself again. The drums beat out the vestiges of violence. As we joined hands in the Circle Dance, a link was formed between myself and all women.

No longer a floater at the department store, I now worked in the office of an eccentric holistic doctor. There, by observation and eavesdropping, I learned that most everyone has some complaint or another from which they seek relief and that there are connections between the health of one's mind and body. One woman was convinced that hair was growing from the palms of her hands (it wasn't), while others were plagued by more conventional problems, such as anemia, sore throats, and stomach aches. A migrant farm worker appeared one afternoon after severely injuring his thumb. I was called in to play nurse. I averted my eyes from the sight of his torn flesh, understanding that but for my sympathetic presence in the examination room, there was nothing I could do. Nor could the doctor change what had happened; he could only dab and stitch. In his own time, the man would heal.

Books like Elizabeth Haich's *Initiation* and Florence Scovil Shinn's *The Game of Life* dropped like magic pennies into the well of my subconscious, disturbing the status quo and creating far-reaching ripples of possibilities. Another such book was *The Secret Oral Teachings* by Alexandra David-Neel and her adopted son, Lama Yongden (who was shown on the cover, wearing a curious pointed hat). By reading these very different accounts of the spiritual realm, I understood that there was more to life (not to mention the hereafter) than I had ever suspected, and yet, paradoxically, in many ways already instinctively knew.

Spiritual journeys are, by their nature, as full of trials and tests as they are rich in rewards. It is said that spirits call the shaman to his work by providing the challenge of an illness or calamity, which is overcome only when appropriately yielded to and thus obeyed. I didn't know enough to yield or obey. Besides, I was no shaman-in-training; I was a moody and impulsive young woman, aware of the moment but not much else. I therefore suffered in a seemingly useless way, the rape ominously slipping into hiding.

Still, it haunted me. My passion was writing, and in a state of near-perpetual inspiration, I would type poem after poem in the sunny back room, sometimes napping afterwards on the soft burgundy sofa. More than once I came suddenly awake from a deep sleep to an extraordinary sound, which can only be described as a buzzing roar, and which hovered around me and seemed to be nothing, if not a manifestation of death.

I didn't see the parallel between this experience, this force or energy which felt evil, otherworldly, and over which I had no control, and Hawaii. I came to recognize it as the personification of my own eventual death, a reminder (perhaps a pestering message) from another dimension. Whatever it was, it was the antithesis of an angel. While I lay trapped in the incoherence of sleep, it caused an unpleasant sinking sensation as it pulled me down and under. Then, just before waking, I would gasp in an effort to release myself, its roar increasing and its spectacle intensifying at the precise moment my eyes opened.

Sometimes, for no obvious reason, I became depressed. I lay in bed for days, paralyzed, trapped in a pit of fear—just as I had been that night. It was as though I were waiting to be rescued. I felt ugly, abandoned, unworthy of love. Who but an all-knowing god could fathom this scene? Certainly not my new boyfriend, lingering hopefully nearby. The language of tears was all that I was capable of speaking.

I was also prone to unruly feelings of agitated dread. First a pressure would build in my throat, making it hard to breathe, then my thinking would become circular, negative, and distorted. Everything seeming worse than it was and with no reprieve likely or possible. I only recently learned that such episodes have a name—anxiety attacks. At least now, when they occur, I can take some comfort in knowing what they are. Yet it is like recalling the name of a poisonous snake when one is in the midst of succumbing to its deadly bite.

In the classic, *Arabian Nights*, Scheherazade invented stories for that great misogynist, the sultan. Under threat of being executed at daybreak, she told of Ali Baba, Aladdin, and Sindbad the Sailor. In the end, she saved herself. As a writer, I, too, told my thousand-and-one tales, my disguised confessions. My pattern was similar: I often wrote during the night, toiling for hours until the birds were singing and the sky lightened. The words were a charm. Writing cleared my soul.

Part II

but I would remember only
how I awoke to familiar fragrance,
late roses, bruised apples;

reality had opened before me,
I had come back;
I retraced the thorny path

H.D.

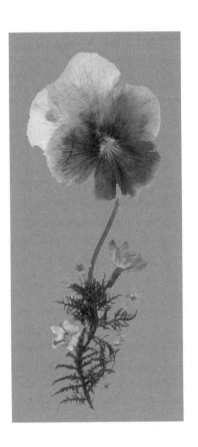

Chain Gang

An incident such as rape transforms itself first in the arena of memory, either destroying or empowering its bearer. Its shadow tests one. I became like a chalice, containing the memory in secret and therefore internalizing it. Although I wanted to speak about what had happened, I was also sure that no one would understand. How could they? And so, silence.

Burdened by this souvenir of evil, preoccupied by the need to keep it hidden from the world, it was hard to feel much ease or self-affinity. Also, since I had let something so terrible happen to me, I could no longer trust myself. This lack of trust migrated to other areas of my life. Uncertainties flourished. The simplest decision, such as buying a dress, took on life-or-death proportions. While it was sometimes strangely liberating in an existential way not to trust anyone or anything (How could I?) it was a painful, debilitating way to live.

I wish that I could say that the memory of that

59

evening is far behind me. Yet even now after a morning of writer's block during which I meditated, lit a candle to invoke the angels, and ate chocolate, I feel those men nearby. They are like the disembodied spirits of a chain gang, ever following me, dangerous but subdued.

Messages

I was warned, if subtly, before my trip to Hawaii. Intuition spoke to me in its suspicious murmur. Its voice was just soft enough so that I could feel justified in ignoring it, though audible enough to impart its message: *Don't go.*

I had heard this voice before, as I'm sure I will again. Sometimes it comes in the form of a split-second vision. Once, when two acquaintances were leaving for a cabin in the woods, I stood in the doorway, "seeing death" around them. Not trusting it or knowing what to do, I simply made a mental note. I later learned that they were asphyxiated during the night by a gas leak.

Another time I was on a bicycle ride with my partner, Pablo, when I "saw" an ambulance. This time, I shouted a warning: "Be careful!" He was cycling fast on the paved path up ahead, weaving erratically, and I felt certain that something was about to happen to him. A moment passed. He must have slowed down or I caught up with him—or both. Suddenly he turned in front of me, his back wheel and my front wheel caught, and I was thrown forward. Time held me in its wings, and when I landed, my chin took the impact. The ambulance which had appeared on my inner horizon was coming for me. I was lucky, they told me later, while stitching me up at the emergency room. Some people died from such injuries.

The next example involves a man named Mr. Blum, who was very devoted to his wife and loved to talk. I was at their home in the suburbs, listening to him describe a luxury cruise they were about to take somewhere. The food! The views! The nightly entertainment! He had written a letter to the ship's captain, asking permission to bring his family and friends (myself included) aboard before setting sail. I felt charmed by this; he was always thinking of others first and not himself.

His new pacemaker monitored his heart as he spoke. He still wore the bandage from his recent operation, but seemed to be adjusting to the device well. Still, I couldn't help but notice how pale he looked. And then I saw it: *Death*. It was the same as before, only this time, I took a moment to say goodbye. I looked deep into his eyes, half-listening to his enthusiastic words about how he was sure the captain would approve his request. Soon after this, he collapsed and died. He never got to go on that cruise.

And then there is Martin. An intelligent man, a gentle soul. I remember a conversation with him in which he shared with me his view of life, that it was important to not race around, but to go slowly, enjoying the smaller moments. Nothing was worth getting too upset about.

I was working at my desk as Martin was in the hall, saying goodbye to Pablo. Martin was going on vacation and I could hear his easygoing voice explaining that he was looking forward to relaxing and riding his bicycle. I wanted to wish him a good trip, but, more than that, I wanted to warn him. For the word "bicycle," despite my personal aversion to it since receiving the stitches on my chin, triggered something. As he continued to talk, I tried but could not get up from my desk. It was as though I were being held back, prevented from interfering.

When the news came that Martin had been in a bicycle accident, that he was in a coma and may not survive, I felt shocked and deeply concerned for him. I also felt ashamed of myself, guilty even. Why hadn't I honored this message? I rationalized that even if I had been able to resist the force-field surrounding my desk, even if I had been able to stand, open the door, and walk down the hall those few steps, he probably wouldn't have listened to me anyway. He had been so set on going, so optimistic.

Somehow, that didn't really help.

In the meantime, Martin lay in a hospital bed. When he finally awakened, he had amnesia and was paralyzed on his left side. He had survived; but his life, which had been irrevocably changed, was still in delicate balance. His journey toward healing was only just beginning.

When I was about five years old, a curious image came to me in the form of a brief yet potent dream. I say "potent" because of all the dreams I've ever had, before or since, this was one that always stayed with me, and I often wondered what, if anything, it meant. At the time, it dominated my world of dreams with its simplicity and power. In the dream, my father was riding a bicycle, and he was blind. Many years passed. Then, around the time my father retired, he was diagnosed with glaucoma, a progressive disease of the eyes which damages the optic nerve and, if left untreated, permanently damages one's sight.

I mention such incidents not to prove or disprove the validity of psychic experiences, but rather to understand something deeper. That they occur is not to be challenged. In all cultures and throughout time, people have listened to their intuition, often as a means of survival. Yet where do these teasing messages come from? Do they originate from within ourselves, or are they the language of angels?

Dr. O.

In the 1990s after many years of silence I finally confessed my story to a therapist, whom I shall call Dr. O. She was a relaxed, likeable woman, who nodded often during our sessions but gave little feedback. It was not an uncommon trait among therapists, this dreamy way they have of listening, drawing out the words by their own peculiar brand of silence, and then, at the end of the forty-five minutes, blithely collecting their fee.

What had begun as couples counseling for Pablo and myself had evolved into individual sessions. During one of these, I mentioned the rape, almost as an afterthought. In the spirit of Scheherazade, I wanted my story, the gloom and heaviness of which I feared might offend, to somehow entertain. I was aware that she had other clients, probably some with worse problems than my own. So, as I began to present a condensed version of that night, it was with politeness. And an eye on the clock.

Her nurturing figure seemed to recede slightly as I

spoke.

For reasons of vanity, it was important to me that I didn't appear too self-pitying. Although inside I felt weak and vulnerable—and often victimized in my daily life—I aimed to appear strong. Given my controlled performance, I only half-expected to experience an epiphany or maybe a few uncontrollable sobs afterwards, so when that didn't happen, I wasn't too disappointed.

She rocked a little in her chair and gently, knowingly, smiled. I think she also may have made a soft "tsk-tsk" with her tongue.

Why is she smiling? I wondered. How can she know? Doesn't she have any probing questions for me? Can't she at least look horrified for half a second?

"It'll always be a part of you. You'll never forget it," she said.

Time passed. I happened to see a program on TV about a prominent politician who had been accused of molesting his female coworkers. To my surprise, Dr. O. was among them. When her turn came to speak, her normally serene face looked pained. I could tell that she had bolstered herself for this interview; she had made the decision to come forward and was now going to be brave and point an accusatory finger at the man who had—. What had he done? Groped her after one-too-many martinis?

A feeling of bitterness clouded my thoughts. Was it just the nagging pull of that wasted eighty dollars? A perverse competitiveness? *My experience was worse than yours.* Or was it the more poignant realization that no one— not therapist, lover, or friend—though they may seek to soothe, shed light, and inspire healing, can ever change what has actually happened. We go on. She was right: It's part of me. I'll never forget it.

Can we ever really know each other's pain? Perhaps not. Yet we can learn to listen well. And that she did.

℟ealing ℂrisis

Secrets make the body toxic. The trauma of rape and the events that surrounded it manifested in my body in various ways. For several years my jaw clicked whenever I chewed; this was a result of being hit. It is still subtly out of alignment. I experience chronic pain on the right side of my neck and back. A female problem required surgery. Recently I was diagnosed with Hashimoto's, an exotic-sounding autoimmune disease in which the thyroid gland thinks that it is being attacked by an outside source and, in turn, self-destructs.

"I want to learn how to heal," I told a friend.

The very next day, on a walk to Golden Gate Park's misty arboretum, I happened upon a psychic fair. After milling about, talking to a few psychics and observing the healings (during which auras were cleaned with an adroit wave of a hand, as though with a feather duster), I decided to attend an angel channeling. Lines of psychics "grounded" the room, while angels supposedly spoke through the six channelers on stage. It was reminiscent of a Victorian parlor game—and more like a revivalist meeting when a woman from the audience became over-emotional—yet I was intrigued by the interesting mix of people and the open atmosphere. I decided to sign up for a beginning meditation class. And so began my brief apprenticeship at the Berkeley Psychic Institute.

Founded in 1972 by the late "Very Right" Reverend Dr. Lewis F. Bostwick, the Institute is located in a former Elks lodge. Walking through its doors, I was met by the knowing eyes of healers, channelers, and clairvoyants. This was a daunting, if illuminating, experience. Immediately I realized that, unlike so many other places in the world, I couldn't hide here.

The cavernous building is haphazardly decorated in a casual, unpretentious way. In the foyer, tropical fish float dreamily in an aquarium. Dozens of folding chairs and a few black vinyl throne-like ones are arranged in the main classroom. "Who needs a healing?" an instructor would ask. Healings were exchanged as naturally as handshakes there. I imagined back-slapping Elks congregating at the bar where clairvoyant students now practice "reading" each other or conducting their secret meetings in the upstairs auditorium-turned-sanctuary.

In *Meditation I*, one learns the basic tools of "psychic kindergarten," which I will not go into here, except to say that they are deceptively simple tools which can render quite powerful results. Students sit "in trance" with their eyes closed and their focus on the center of their heads. One important lesson of psychic kindergarten is that of "finding one's amusement," hence the spontaneous, often contagious laughter of the clairvoyant students. Yet I would have a difficult time laughing about what was to happen next.

I had completed the six-week course and was now enrolled in two simultaneous classes: *Women's Intuition* and *Healing I.* Back and forth I traveled on BART (Bay Area Rapid Transit) through that long underwater tube which connects San Francisco with the East Bay. It was an especially stressful time. I had over-committed to various projects, my home life was miserable, and I had been asked to give a series of public talks about a guidebook I'd written—never mind that I had no public speaking experience and was terrified. My life seemed like one big learning curve.

The Institute's director was an Australian named Wayne. He wore rose-colored glasses (the rose was the Institute's mascot flower; perhaps he did this out of respect) and, from the back, his gleaming shaved head resembled a crystal ball. During our first *Healing I* class, he stood before us in his neon orange tee shirt and baggy jeans with the cuffs turned up, looking both strong and vulnerable, eager and reserved. He told a story about the first time he had ever felt an aura and soon had us walking slowly about the room, hands extended, trying to sense the differences in energy between chair and wall, as well as with each other. There was also some alarming talk of "psychic surgeons," those people who can pluck disease (often in the form of a reddish-black egg dripping blood) from one's body. I didn't believe a word of it.

In subsequent classes, we practiced healing each other. Sometimes I could feel a subtle shift as my partner's hand passed over, circled, or gently raked what was perceived to be my aura; it was the same when I, in turn, passed my hand over theirs. Such intimate attention, often wordless, in which one looks beyond appearances into the spirit within is rare among strangers. That alone was healing.

A few weeks went by. The focus of this class was chakras, energy centers from the base of the spine to the top of the head in which blockages, and thus disease, can occur. Wayne was discussing the second, or sacral, chakra located in the pelvic area when I became aware of intense pain in my groin. "Excuse me!" I whispered, as I darted from the class. Thinking that my problem was a simple urinary tract infection, I returned to class only to leave again, return, and leave again. Soon I was doubled up inside the BART restroom. The problem was I couldn't urinate.

Hours passed. The pressure was building. I hopped on one foot and then another. I prayed. At one point, BART workers congregated outside the locked door, discussing chitlings and other soul food. From time to time there were a few polite knocks.

Then, not knowing what else to do, I made a run for it down the escalator and onto the arriving train, where I desperately clutched a book and pretended to read, all the while quivering and breathing deeply. The woman seated next to be must have thought I was insane. Time passed agonizingly slowly, as it always does when one is in pain.

A friend eventually took me to the emergency room where I was fitted with a catheter, which relieved the pressure of my "urethral spasm." Finally I had the luxury of wondering, *What's happening to me?*

While lying on the hard white table, I had a realization. One of the psychic tools is a grounding cord, which allegedly extends from the base of the spine to the center of the earth, and through which unwanted energy is released. I glanced at the plastic tube extending daintily out of my body down into the pan. Then I remembered when this illness had struck—during the chakra class. Coincidence?

A few days later, these words came to me while I was driving myself (catheter and all) to the first of my public talks: *By healing it [the rape], I'm allowing it to empower me.* My healing crisis—or "growth period" as they call it—was a way *through* the pain. If I could emerge intact from the other side, I would be that much stronger.

$\mathcal{Y}$oga

"Yoga is about finding space in your body," the instructor says in her melodic British accent. "It's about breath." She gracefully moves among us as we lie in the Corpse Pose on our purple mats.

I close my eyes and tell myself to relax. Something in me resists. Ever since writing about the rape, I have been plagued by paranoia. Where are those two men now? In prison probably, or reformed, recovered, middle-aged with regrets. Perhaps they are dead. That I escaped with my anonymity was my saving grace, my only protection. If these words are ever read by them, that will be lost.

I consider asking a friend who has become a private detective to check their whereabouts, but even that is traumatic. Stating their actual names makes them more real, brings them into the present moment.

As the instructor talks about *prana*, the life force, I try to feel it coursing through me. I breathe slowly in and out. In the stillness of the room my arm and leg muscles

73

begin to soften. I can almost sense a rising peace within me, hinting at enlightenment.

Almost. Feeling exposed and vulnerable as she paces past, any potential bliss falls away. I am reminded of the drowned Ophelia of Millais's painting—lying clothed in the dark water, moored by crow flowers and daisies, her face expressionless, hands limp—which is how I must have looked that night.

The instructor bends down beside me. *"Breathe!"* she whispers.

And so I gasp, struggling to reclaim and inhabit *my* body.

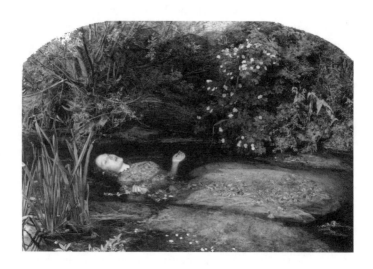

Somersaults

It is a blustery day in Hampstead, London. The roads are dark and slick, and the shop windows reflect an alternate universe in which we are not all strangers but in some way kindred, recognizable as actually belonging together in this moment, entrenched as we are in the here and now. The trees, whipped by wind, look shaken and shell-shocked, their bare limbs lifted to the sky as though in surrender.

As I walk, I think about how the rape was (and yet was not) an isolated event in my personal chronology. Although the shock of it alone does isolate it from everything that came before and after it, there are aspects of it that match too well the thematic shades of my life. I wonder, too, why so many women, by virtue of our gender, experience similar forms of victimization.

When I was very young, I regarded a neighbor-boy's penis (the first I'd ever seen) while standing in a particularly enchanted part of my backyard. How small and shriveled it was—and how mysterious! It represented far more than I, at five, was capable of understanding. That same boy would later force me to lie down in the middle of the road, as though I were a lady tied to train tracks, and he a bandit. Before running off, he warned me not to move. I was that still little figure just beyond the blind curve where Duchess the beagle had been struck dead by a milk truck.

Another time, a friend's father urged me to pull down my pants on the pretense of touching my scar. He then took me to see his newly remodeled bathroom, which was decorated by many small polished stones which supposedly became even more beautiful when water fell on them. I remember feeling in awe of the stones, and, though nothing actually happened, wary of his too-eager smile. There is something about innocence which tempts certain anguished souls to try to destroy it.

When I was about twelve, after my piano lesson (during which I had stumbled through *Moonlight Sonata*), a man in a car giddily exposed himself to me. The policeman who later turned up in our kitchen to interview me made a mockery of the event by being *too* tactful; it was as though he were reading from a poor script. Once I came across a man masturbating in a public place and—perhaps because of these previous injustices—scolded him.

The experience of "date rape" (which I define as something entirely different and distinct from regular rape by virtue of one's relationship with that person and the degree of life-threatening violence involved) occurred when I was a coffee-shop waitress and made the foolish mistake of dating the cook. I mention these sordid episodes to give the reader a sense of context to the rape: My life as a girl and a woman has been, at turns, absurd and humiliating.

Yet I have also been blessed with relationships with remarkable men and have thankfully known love of the sweet and requited variety. I like most men; I have even loved a few too much. Still, I'm often perplexed and disheartened by the historically violent ways of the male of our species. Never mind that so many of them are afraid of commitment and, when lost, won't ask for directions.

Why do they rape? Why do they kill?

Fleeing the cold, I duck into Waterstone's bookshop. There, nestled between other more inviting books, is *A Natural History of Rape*. My first reaction is to recoil. The word "rape" seems to float ominously toward me. With trepidation, I turn to the first chapter.

By one intuitive and relevant definition, rape is copulation resisted to the best of the victim's ability unless such resistance would probably result in death or serious injury of the victim or in death or injury to individuals the victim commonly protects.

The authors—two men, Thornhill and Palmer— have taken an evolutionary and biological approach to the subject. They have provided theories and statistics that explain man's historical, sexual coercion of women. Their focus is on the ultimate cause of such behavior rather than purely circumstantial or cultural reasons.

Taking this objective "long view" on such an intensely personal subject can be off-putting, at least it is for me. Yet something draws me in; it is the promise of finding information to ease my anguish, which in recent years has grown all the more powerful. I need to understand my place in this drama in order to relinquish some of my shame. And so I read on, skeptical, but open. The words of academics have a soothing, if mollifying, effect.

I am startled to learn that rape does not occur only between humans.

Experiments reveal that male scorpionflies prefer to provide mates with nuptial food gifts...and that they rape only when they cannot provide such gifts.

This fact I contemplate with some compassion, picturing the bewildered, frantic female and the desire-driven male. So we humans are not alone. Even insects, supposedly blind to what drives them (though who really knows?) are compelled to repeat the same tragic behavior, to suffer through these acts of desire, domination, and violation. Perhaps we can't help ourselves. It would seem that we are all caught up in something greater and more profound than our individual lives can comfortably accommodate.

Are we as superior to other species as we would like to think? Keeping in mind the scorpionfly's nuptial gifts, one need only consider human mating rituals in which the man buys the woman a drink and/or dinner with the expectation of sexual favors returned.

This dance between male and female is as complex as it is heart-wrenchingly routine. Females apparently learn something called "avoidance behavior." The female waterstrider does somersaults to thwart the male's rape

78

attempt.

No somersaults could have saved me that night.

The authors went on to give other justifications for male aggression, causing me to wonder about the subliminal stirrings, the imbalances of want/need and attraction/repulsion which link us to other species. Maybe it's all true, I think, as I slowly turn the pages. But like a dog who is attuned to a higher, more piercing frequency, I can hear only screams.

$\mathcal{P}$ersephone & $\mathcal{D}$emeter

If you relate to my story, you are like many other women (and girls) who have been betrayed, humiliated, controlled, or attacked in some way. Every two minutes, on average, a woman is raped in America. Each year, approximately 250,000 women are the victims of rape, attempted rape, or sexual assault.[1] Less than one in three of the 17.7 million American women who have suffered such an experience ever report it (RAINN). In Britain, specifically England and Wales, 60,000 women are raped in a year and over 750,000 women claim to have been raped since they were aged sixteen. Eighty per cent of these incidents go unreported (British Crime Survey). The situation is worse for women in the "unliberated" world.[2]

This has been our shared legacy. Think of the great gulf of silence kept by those who were, and are, too frightened or ashamed to revisit the unthinkable, to describe the indescribable. Shame is a broken umbrella; it serves no one.

Persephone & Demeter

Ours is like the story of Persephone, who was once a lighthearted maiden. Her days were spent in the company of nymphs, gathering wildflowers. In the ancient Greek myth, she was seized by Hades, god of the underworld, and taken to his realm where she was raped by him and forced to live as his partner, becoming the goddess of the dead.

While Persephone's mother, Demeter, goddess of plants and fertility, searches for her lost daughter, the earth, like her heart, becomes desolate and barren. Only in spring does Hades allow Persephone to be reunited with Demeter on the condition—which is ensured by her eating a pomegranate seed—that she always return to the underworld.

Many of us spend a lifetime hiding in the underworld. It is a murky place full of secrets, confusion, and misdirected rage. Like Persephone, we may emerge from it; but, if only in the heartbeat of a memory, we seem always bound to return.

I write these words on my mother's eightieth birthday. Like Demeter, she would have been just as desperate to rescue me from my plight. But I never told her (or my father) what happened to me in Hawaii. When I returned to San Francisco, I waited a few weeks while the bruise healed and then called to say that I was back, that I'd had a great time in paradise. By protecting her, I reasoned, I was, in turn, protecting myself. Maybe if she hadn't been so strong a force (at times an emotional wild card, sure that the worst was always about to happen and even when it didn't, quick to overreact), maybe if I'd felt that I could count on her as a source of comfort and consolation... And yet, just as Persephone needed her mother as ally, I also needed mine.

So as she repeatedly told me her tales of early life in rural Montana, of no running water or electricity, of footprints of Indians in the snow, the trauma of being in a spelling bee (which she won), the time her brothers locked her in a shed and a bat got tangled in her hair, train whistles in the night, killing a snake with a hoe, I reciprocated with silence. Although I'm sure she sensed the changes in me, the maiden lost, unlike Demeter, she just didn't know *how* to find me.

---

[1]Men and boys are also raped and sexually assaulted, though it is not as common.

[2]Honor killings, in which the male members of a woman's family are duty-bound to end her life if she has brought shame on them by her actual or perceived immoral behavior, and female genital mutilation, which is prevalent in over thirty countries around the world, are two examples.

Ruby

The now-ancient scene repeated itself in flashbacks—two men, a knife. This holographic vision superimposed itself on the mundane events of my life. A sudden noise or a violent scene on TV would prompt their reappearance. And there they'd be: floating before me as I boiled potatoes, potted geraniums, or read a book. They were like ghosts, lost and wandering; they sought me out. I never knew when they might appear. As they hunched near me, drawing the blade, I wondered, *How can others not also see this?*

Finally it became too much. My friend Roger—boisterous, spontaneous, and with his own unique brand of *joie de vivre*—was the marketing director of a small publishing company in Berkeley. I sensed in him a kindred spirit. After knowing him only six months, prompted by intense, recurrent flashbacks, I decided to reveal to him what had happened in Hawaii. It was a story that I had not told to family, or to many of my closest friends.

It was a dry, hot summer day, the air charged with electricity. Roger and I were sitting outside on a wooden deck, relaxing in lawn chairs. I was drinking white wine, and he was smoking a cigar. Ruby, the quadriplegic dog whom he was looking after while her owners were on vacation, lay nearby.

"Begin," he said.

"I can't. I'm afraid."

"What of?"

"I guess I'm afraid that I'll cry so much, I won't be able to stop."

"So, cry."

"I don't want to."

He took another puff, nonchalantly blowing smoke rings into the air. Ruby whined.

"Okay," I said, after a moment. "Here goes."

My voice sounded tinny and flat, as though it came from a distance and was not my own. Gradually, more words followed, until I had led my listener to a point of no return.

"And then?"

I paused. I didn't want to say the word "rape."

Sensing my discomfort, Roger found a feather in the flower-bed and placed it in my hair. I felt like a squaw now, amused and empowered. It's moments like these when a laugh can turn to tears. (But I didn't cry then—I still haven't.) Roger pushed the fingers of his hands together, playing the part of therapist, and said, "Continue."

"I was *raped*," I said.

He waited a beat, then glanced at me. "That's terrible. You shouldn't feel ashamed, you know."

"I shouldn't?"

He flicked ash from his cigar. "Of course not."

By the end of my story, I noticed something odd. In my mind's eye, Hyena and Dark One had receded. Rather than lurking menacingly over the bed, where they usually appeared in flashbacks, they now stood farther back, near the doorway.

"And so that's what happened," I concluded, with a sudden rush of strength and clarity. I got up and stretched. Something had changed in the telling.

That night, Ruby the dog took ill. We didn't notice at first. We had come inside to cook dinner, leaving Ruby in her prone position on the deck. She had seemed her usual self, an elderly quadriplegic dog who was unable to move more than her head and her tail. "Good girl!" we had said, patting her. Her watery brown eyes possessed a depth not found in those of most dogs—or most people.

Roger was of the belief that she should be "put down," that it was the most humane thing to do considering her condition. Ruby's owners may have agreed, but they were attached to her, perhaps overly so. For years Ruby had lay in the basement, listening to classical music, or was carefully lifted and carried in someone's arms, like a queen upon a sedan chair. She had become an icon.

When I had first met Ruby, I couldn't help but kneel down and stroke her head, which subtly bobbed and swayed in greeting. I wanted to help her. I wanted to see her run and fetch and do all the normal things dogs do, but she couldn't. All she could do was offer her heartbreaking expression of hopefulness. And of course that was what melted one—that fragile, useless body overtaken by the oddly joyful power of her canine spirit.

Ruby had much to teach me in the way of attitude. She had no self-pity or resentment for her condition, not even a trace of bitterness from what I could tell. Ruby was in the moment. Whether this was a full-fledged experience of enlightenment like Buddhists strive for or her own form of emotional negotiation with her fate, I don't know. Maybe she was there simply because she had no other choice.

Roger and I were in the kitchen, cooking risotto. Now that I had told him my story, I began to feel awkward. What did he think of me? Should I not have told him? But it was too late. I couldn't take the words back; they had settled between us, were already part of our history. Soon we fell into a rhythm of chopping vegetables (I automatically cringed when I saw the knife), waltzing between sink and stove, laughing and drinking more wine. Oh, how I welcomed such mundane talk after my confession!

Roger likes everything to be just so. He had set the table with care and lit two candles. The soundtrack from the film *Buena Vista Social Club* was playing softly in the background. We were between bites, marveling at our meal, when we heard the first whimper. This was not unusual for Ruby, but there was a tinge more distress, so Roger, a father of two with a strong paternal instinct, set down his fork and stomped out to the deck to investigate.

"She's panting," he shouted.

I got down on all fours alongside him and studied Ruby's heaving chest. Dog breath overshadowed the delicate flavor of the risotto. It was always difficult to know just what Ruby was feeling or what she needed. We shouted in her ear as though she were deaf, which she might have been. "Are you too hot? Do you want some water?"

Although it was getting dark, I could see that her eyes looked bloodshot. Saliva drooled from her mouth, pooling between her paws. The shaking continued. Something was wrong.

"Up we go!" said Roger. He carted her into the dining room, laid her gently on her fluffy pink rug, and nudged her water dish closer.

We resumed eating, occasionally glancing over at Ruby, like two worried parents.

"It's the Rube!" he exclaimed.

We waited for her tail to wag, but it didn't.

"Rube?"

"Why is she trembling so?" I asked him.

Again, Roger set down his fork. "I've seen her shaking before, but never like this." He ran to her and placed his hand across her chest. "Feel her heart," he said. "It's beating so fast, I can't even count it."

While Roger made calls—first to a nearby animal hospital, then to a nurse friend, and on and on—I sat with Ruby. I had no doubt that she would die that night. How could she survive? She had been panting for hours with no reprieve. Her heartbeats were those of a dog who had been chased for hours through unfamiliar woods. Ruby kept raising her head and looking at me with an urgent, dazed expression. I held her paw. "She's still trembling," I called to Roger. "Her tongue is dry." It was strange to have earlier unburdened myself about Hawaii and now to be seeing a dog through to the other side.

And then I saw it: Wasn't that me, lying on the bed, afraid, shaking uncontrollably, almost dying? It was as though I were comforting, or even rescuing, myself.

Ruby didn't die. Apparently it was just a seizure of some sort. Her body was breaking down. Soon she wouldn't even be able to lift her head.

Months passed. Roger and I were talking on the phone, gossiping, jumping from subject to subject, when finally he mentioned Ruby. "They're putting her down tonight," he said.

I drew in a breath. "Poor Ruby!" I'll say a prayer for her, I thought. Later, I looked at the starry sky and wished her well, wherever she was going. I imagined her as happy and healthy as a new puppy. She deserved such an existence—even better—after all she'd been through.

When I next spoke to Roger, I inquired about Ruby's owners. How were they coping? Had they recovered from the loss?

"They couldn't do it," he said. "They got as far as the vet's, carried her in, said their goodbyes, and then they broke down and brought her back home."

"I guess it wasn't her time."

"No," he sighed. "The Rube's still with us."

Walking Wounded

The experience of rape, if viewed in a spiritual light, can offer hard-won lessons. As the Chinese say: "Crisis equals opportunity." Yet traumatic events linger.

Post-traumatic Stress Disorder (PTSD) is really just a fancy name for one's natural response to profound and unexpected shock and the associated symptoms which are, in fact, normal reactions to abnormal events. It can result after experiencing or even witnessing traumatic and/or life-threatening events such as rape, child abuse, war, torture, airplane crashes, and natural disasters.

It is regrettable that such buzzwords have the effect of distancing us or disguising their true meaning by their formality. It is as though the afflicted are herded together under a sign that says "PTSD" or "ADD" (Attention Deficit Disorder) or some other jumbling of the alphabet, and then, once categorized, forgotten about. The very language itself obstructs understanding. It misses the hidden depth behind those labels.

For it is a world peopled by the walking wounded. Some limp along, while others feel their way blind, and still others hide their wounds even from themselves. The trauma remains, influencing the present moment with its past power.[3]

The physical and emotional symptoms of PTSD are extreme, disruptive, and unpredictable. They include anxiety, distress, and irritability, as well as opposite feelings of detachment and emotional numbness as one tries to avoid the pain of the experience. Some people work excessively to keep the upsetting memories at bay, while others turn to drugs and/or alcohol. Sufferers may become depressed, have trouble concentrating, and experience sleep problems such as insomnia and nightmares. By day, they can be easily startled. They may also have disturbing memories and flashbacks which may be triggered by events in the outer world.

For instance, watching the evening news can be risky for me. Suddenly, without warning, there will be a chilling report of rape or some related crime, and images of the victim (who may have survived—or not), and the perpetrator (who may have been caught—or not) will appear on the screen. The immediate alarm and grief and fear felt as a sharp pinprick to my consciousness is intensified by its random, unexpected nature. The woman, often unnamed, who has been violently acted-upon thus loses her identity, becomes all women, any woman, and therefore me. To the public, she is simply misfortune's icon. She has received her unwanted, unenviable initiation. Although she may heal, she will never be the same. It is no wonder, given her new victim status, that she feels ashamed.

The perpetrator is often shown caught off-guard at his most wicked and vulnerable. His eyes contain his crime. Not wanting to be apprehended by yet another memory, I always try not to meet his gaze.

Films are just as bad. The scenes of rape often seem contrived, melodramatic, and unbelievable. There is not just one way to be raped. It does not always happen quickly. The woman does not always scream. She does not always cry hysterically, uncontrollably, or know what she feels (if anything) afterwards.

"Whenever we give up, leave behind, and forget too much, there is always the danger that the things we have neglected will return with added force," wrote Jung.

Sometimes, out of the blue, when the two return to haunt me, it is as though they have been waiting quietly off-stage for some unknown cue, so eager are they to terrorize me all over again. They move with the same menacing footsteps, they speak the same threatening language. As though caught under a strobe light, their faces are revealed to me only as cryptic snapshots.

With any of these triggers, I feel an inappropriate, but instinctive need to protect myself. I freeze like a cat whose spine draws into a bow. I become withdrawn, anxious, or irritable—or worse, a combination of the three. Each time my trust is unnecessarily challenged, a vital part of me is used up in the process.

Here is an example of the kind of innocent occasion that can undo me. A lone palm tree, glimpsed out the window of a B&B in Campbeltown, Scotland, prompted a nightmare, from which I woke up gasping. Not all palm trees have this effect.[4] But whenever I see one, or see its image on a piece of fabric or even read the words "palm tree oil" on a label, I react, if only to experience a numb recognition that palm tree = Hawaii = rape = danger. It is a loop of thought, which my mind dumbly follows.

Other triggers: My mother's pineapple upside-down cake. Orchids. Coconut shampoo. All of which I actually like, by the way. Driving past a brilliant yellow field recently, I was horrified to hear my friend call out, "Oh, look at the lovely rapeseed flowers!"

Of course, it was not always like this. Once, when I was in elementary school, we had a Hawaiian festival. After weeks of preparation, the classroom was transformed into a rickety paradise. There was a sense of playful anticipation as *poi* was served (a grey paste of fermented taro root) and we girls, wearing leis and grass skirts, performed the hula. I can still remember the graceful swaying moves, complete with hand gestures, as we sang:

> *It's not the islands fair*
> *That are calling to me*
> *It's not the balmy air*
> *Nor the tropical sea*
> *It's just a little brown gal*
> *In a little grass skirt*
> *In a little grass shack in Hawai'i.*

When someone has just returned from a trip to "the islands" (not an uncommon occurrence in California), it is only natural to inquire about the weather, where they stayed, and what they did. I never want to know. The difficulty is not being able to explain why. Or,

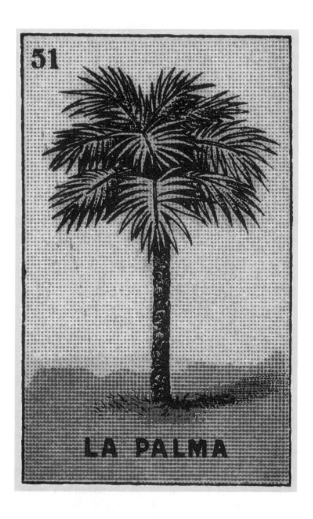

overcompensating for the fact that I am trapped in the conversation, I might become *too* interested in their trip. I'll hear myself say, "Oh, yes, Hawaii—what an *amazing* place!"

It hurts to pretend. Much energy is spent suppressing trauma and diverting truth. A leaflet by the Traumatic Stress Clinic explains the dichotomy of this disorder:

The symptoms of PTSD are thought to arise as the person naturally tries to push the event out of their mind but finds that it continues to intrude. Thus they alternate between trying to come to terms with what has happened and not wanting to think about the traumatic event.

Even when we don't think about it, we are still affected. The trauma is in our bones. Some women, long after the rape itself, feel unclean. They compulsively keep taking baths and changing clothes in order to purify themselves. Rape's "violation of intimacy" also affects relationships, making it difficult to trust again. Perhaps that is why I never married, why I have no children. Was I robbed, I wonder, not only of my innocence, but also of a path in life?

Depression is a common symptom of trauma survivors, sabotaging the health of one's mind, body, and spirit. It manifested in me as intense hopelessness, crying jags, and difficulty making decisions. At times, when the undecipherable pain became too great, the act of breathing itself was imbued with dread, and I wondered if, like Virginia Woolf (herself a survivor of sexual trauma and the trauma of World War II), I might place a stone in my pocket, find my own River Ouse, and drown myself. Fortunately that didn't happen.

In the world of PTSD, depression is just a starting-point. If one doesn't acknowledge that something bad has happened and seek help, it can progress. One's life can be changed, a second time, by the impact of these unresolved symptoms.

---

[3]See Chapter Two, "Consciousness: The Way Out of Pain," in Eckhart Tolle's *The Power of Now: A Guide to Spiritual Enlightenment.*

[1]In fact, the palm tree is commonly regarded as a noble tree. From the upright column of its trunk radiates a crown of wispy, featherlike fronds. In biblical times, its branches were carried in processions, then saved for good luck and protection. Jesus' cross was made of four woods, one of which was palm (the part of the cross to which His hands were nailed). Christians traditionally carry palm fronds (or in England, pussy willows) on Palm Sunday. Angels were once believed to use palm fronds to carry souls on their way to heaven. Pilgrims often walked with palm tree staffs. The palm is a symbol of peace, martyrdom, victory. Pointing straight to heaven, this ancient tree demonstrates the spiritual principle of verticality, connecting man with the divine. It represents spiritual triumph.

Spider

   While writing about Post-traumatic Stress Disorder, I happen to glance up at the ceiling at a spider. I am not fond of spiders, but I can't kill them. They seem so alert and all-knowing, if a little devious. Usually when I find a spider at home, after much trepidation, I manage to capture it in a jar. I release it outside, often in the garden. This involves carrying the jar down flights of stairs, then trying to coax the balled, vaguely camouflaged spider out onto a vine of ivy. Other times, I give the spider a thrill by floating it out the window. The entire process always upsets me. Although I am terrified of the spider, I always wish it well and pray that it won't return.

   But this spider is too high up to catch. It's on the ceiling. I try to think of it as a spirit. Grandmother Spider was a benevolent healer, according to the Native Americans. This doesn't seem to help. I can feel the spider's eerie gaze bearing down upon me.

   I creep across the room and stand under it to get a

better look, hoping it won't think to suddenly drop down on its bungee-web. I can feel my heart pounding. My breaths are short. My thoughts race. Maybe I should find a ladder? Then I think of the elderly woman I once saw in the emergency room who had fallen off a ladder and broken her arm, thanks to an unwelcome spider. How will I be able to sleep while it makes its stealthy way across the ceiling, into the next room, down the wall, onto me? Because I can sense its crafty logic.

I blow, hoping the gust will startle it toward the window. There is no response.

Stubborn.

How can I write? Every time I have a thought, a feeling of dread draws my attention back to the ceiling. Nonetheless, I struggle along, blaming it for my writer's block.

The next morning, I remember about the spider. I'm hoping it won't have traveled much. I see it's still there. That's a relief. Then I take another look. I squint. Wait! It's not a spider! Strange, I was so sure.

And then it occurs to me: This is exactly what Post-traumatic Stress Disorder is all about: perceiving a threat when, in fact, there is none—and then wholeheartedly reacting to it. It's exhausting. It changes everything. It makes vicious, maniacal spiders out of motes of dust.

$\mathcal{A}$ngel of $\mathcal{M}$ercy

A few days after Christmas, 1999, I found a man collapsed in the underground Muni station in San Francisco. No one was helping him, and the crowd mentality was persuading me to do the same. Besides, I was late and in a hurry. I had grown accustomed to fixing my gaze elsewhere when confronted by the distressing sight of a homeless person.

Yet something about this man seemed different. For one, he was wearing a scruffy wool suit and nice shoes. There was no styrofoam cup nearby, no cardboard sign with the words, "Hungry. Please help." He wasn't begging; in fact, he hadn't moved at all. I studied his chest to see if he was breathing. Was he dead? I took a step back.

A little circle of emptiness had formed around myself and the man, an invisible barrier that prevented anyone else from becoming involved or feeling even a glimmer of humanity. I bent down and spoke to him.

"Are you all right?" It was a stupid question, because

obviously he wasn't.

I should point out that I am no saint. I am just as selfish—probably more so—than anyone else. I just felt an inexplicable connection with this man. I wanted to help.

"Can you hear me?"

There was a muffled sound, and his eyes slowly opened. They were the most incredible aquamarine blue and they seemed to be lit from deep inside. Despite his semi-inebriated state, they focused on me kindly and knowingly, much the way Clarence the angel's did on Jimmy Stewart in the film, *It's a Wonderful Life.*

"Oh..." He raised his head of tousled white hair, then slid back down.

I kneeled on the hard marble floor as trains whished past. I was going to be late, but it didn't matter. Besides, he was taking my hand. I couldn't turn away.

It came to pass that he told me some of his life story. He had been in World War II. Friends of his had died. He seemed to feel guilty about that.

Post-Traumatic Stress Disorder, I thought. Here it was 1999; the war had been over for over fifty years, and yet, to him, it was still vivid. He probably saw himself lying in a foxhole somewhere, wounded. It was as though he had never recovered. With a pang of recognition, I saw myself in him: an ordinary, well-meaning person who had inadvertently been taken to hell and back and whose fragile negotiations with peace and joy had since often failed. Wasn't a part of me still trapped in that room in Hawaii, while I pretended otherwise?

"It's not your fault. You did the right thing," I heard myself say. I didn't know where the words came from or if they were even right.

He looked at me with those eyes again, that brilliant flash of blue.

At one point, a Muni worker approached. By then the old man had drifted off, but I was staying near, sure that he would soon remember something else and wake up again. She gave him a little kick. A kick! "Sir, you're on the floor. Don't you want to get up?"

"Awwwrrrhhh." He sighed and grunted, propping himself up on an elbow. A discussion of old show tunes followed. He was feeling better now. The Muni worker had arranged for an ambulance; it was time for me to go. When I started to interrupt him, he blinked at me intently, as though in disbelief.

"Do I know you?" he asked. He leaned closer and smiled. "Are you...an angel of mercy?"

"No," I said, embarrassed. "I don't think so."

Then my train arrived. I said good-bye, hurried aboard, and took a seat. Glancing out the window, I thought that if anyone were an angel, it was the one with the halo of white hair.

Cookies

Vanessa, my old friend and roommate in San Francisco, now lives in northern California with her second husband, Tom. Their home, a spectacular Victorian, is always open to friends and relatives, as well as the occasional stranger. It is place of good food and celebration. Although she had invited me to visit her there often over the years, I had always refused. It just seemed too painful to see her again and to not acknowledge what had happened in Hawaii. But now with my trip to London planned (along with the fact that I was running out of excuses) I wanted to do just that. I also wanted to confront her about how she had never really "been there" for me during the rape's aftermath, instead cheerfully carrying on with her life while I was struggling to find my footing.

When I arrived, her youngest daughter stood in the doorway. She was only two. With her tiny, terrycloth robe, angelic, curly blonde hair, and mischievous expression, she looked like a miniature Vanessa. The real

Vanessa was doing some last-minute grocery shopping, so Tom led me inside.

Vanessa, Tom, and I had all gone to high school together. We'd been neighbors in "the circle." Each of them had first married other people before coming together as a couple. It was strange seeing him in his new role as the lord of the manor.

I remembered how many years ago I'd stayed overnight at Tom's house, sleeping in the same room as his pet python. I don't especially like snakes, but it was in a cage so I assumed that it would be no threat. As I tried to fall asleep, I could hear the rustle as the snake flexed its muscular body. The next morning, Tom wandered into the room holding in his cupped hand the unfortunate mouse who was to be the snake's breakfast. He frowned. "Oops." He had forgotten to put the lid on the cage. At any point during the night, the snake could have slithered out. Fortunately it didn't.

Perhaps it was also strange for him to see me. There was a pause as the years fast-forwarded, and we each thought of what to say. "How's your mom?" I asked, realizing as I did that I had never really thanked her for taking me to that counseling session, sitting beside me with an air of nonjudgmental support. Aside from Henry, she was the one other person who really *had* been there for me.

We made small talk; I admired a lamp. And then in walked Vanessa.

"Hi, honey!" There she was again—joyful, exuberant—as she deposited her groceries and led me up and down the polished stairs, pointing out various artifacts and treasures. I wanted to ask (but didn't) if her cherished ceramic bowl—once her only possession—was mixed somewhere among them.

I couldn't help noticing that while I had isolated myself as a writer, living a bohemian lifestyle to support that dream, Vanessa had acquired an incredible home. The towering Christmas tree alone, decorated with its sparkling crystals, was enough to drive a pang of envy through my heart. Plus two children and a devoted man. *Two* men, if one counted her first husband who lived, quite amicably, in the carriage house behind them. Not only that, but inspired by her own past experience as a ward of the court, she was intent on adopting a little girl named Betty and had launched a campaign to do so, generating dozens of letters (which she showed me) all attesting to Vanessa's exemplary character. "What's another mouth to feed?" she said in that generous, headstrong way of hers.

I felt stunted in her presence. I could barely deal with myself, let alone another person. It seemed my life had been on hold, while hers had manifested both personal and material riches.

I waited until after her assorted dinner guests had come and gone and the friendly boarder had gone to sleep to bring up the subject. We were standing at the kitchen sink washing and drying dishes under the enormous, stuffed moose head, whose glassy eyes, while they looked elsewhere, seemed quietly aware of us. "Do you remember about Hawaii?" I asked her, as I carefully placed an expensive glass upon the spotless shelf.

She looked at me squarely. "You mean the rape?"

I started to say what I'd planned, but even as the

words left my mouth, they seemed trite. Besides, it suddenly occurred to me that she *had* been there. It was I who hadn't been there for myself.

"I can see how you'd be upset. It was a life-threatening experience," she offered.

So she understood: Rape was about more than sex. That insight, in itself, was a gift. I felt relieved, even buoyed, and was about to say more.

"Hungry?" she asked. She popped a cookie jar under my nose and opened the lid, the scent of cinnamon wafting out. "Homemade. Take your pick. Chocolate or oatmeal-raisin." Clearly, that one incident that had preoccupied me for years didn't hold the same power over her. To my disappointment, we sat together at her round oak table, eating and dunking, and the conversation moved on. After all, she had married Tom, our old high school friend. She had had his child. And her first husband was in the carriage house.

Maybe Hawaii had never happened. Maybe I had only imagined coming home that day with a bruised face.

"Remember Bounce and Stella?"

"Remember Ting-a-Ling?"

These were old pets of hers, two great danes and a Siamese cat. Then, recalling the escapade when we had hid in the girl's restroom, drinking Cointreau, she got that mischievous look. "Remember the fire drill?"

Doubling over as we laughed, we frantically waved our hands, trying not to spit out milk. It was just too funny. Oh, how we howled! Now, if only for a little while, we were teenagers again.

Butterfly Effect

My father used to tell me a story about a butterfly who, by the flutter of her wings, affected one thing and then another, eventually producing a change that was felt on the other side of the world. I remember looking to the sky and frowning as I took in the implications of a butterfly having such power. How could this be? As my young mind struggled to understand the truth of what he'd said, something shifted within me, resulting in a different way of seeing. So life was one great, ever-changing field of possibilities. I later learned that his story was not a story at all. It was a principle of chaos theory called the Butterfly Effect, in which anything can affect anything else, resulting in "order masquerading as randomness."

My father also liked to recite Sir Walter Scott's "O what a tangled web we weave, when first we practice to deceive!" Here the butterfly's role in altering the course of things was usurped by truth's rival, the lie. Just as the flight of a lone butterfly across a meadow had the potential to wreak havoc by causing a storm somewhere else, apparently thoughts and words, in the form of lies (including, I supposed, "white" lies), could also do damage. His were moral messages: Don't lie. And watch what you do, for it has an effect on others.

I thought of my father's parental instructions when I decided to write this book. I didn't have the luxury of much forethought, swept up as I was by flashbacks and the impulse to confess in words, or else I probably wouldn't have dared. Like most of the turning points in my life, there was about it a ragged sense of inevitability. Preparing inwardly had taken me years; now I faced the equal challenge of doing it.

Before coming to London, I met with Henry (who had wired me money in Hawaii) and his family—mother, sister, aunt, and Camille, his girlfriend—at the St. Francis, a posh, Union Square hotel. It was our annual holiday tea, the last of the millennium, which added significance to the occasion.

"What will you be doing in London?" the mother asked.

"Oh, writing," I said.

The sister, an expert in negotiations at the United Nations in Washington, D.C., turned to me, dabbed her mouth, and said, "Writing what?"

Rape is not a good topic for tea-time conversation. And yet, owing to the fact that I only saw these busy people once a year, if that, small talk wouldn't suffice. "More tea, anyone?" I asked, stalling.

It worked, almost. Then, over the cascading harp music, I heard her ask again.

"Sorry, I just can't discuss it," I answered lamely.

The sister batted her eyes at me ingenuously. This was a woman who had lived in Beirut during the bombing. She knew about trauma.

"Just let us read it when you're finished," the mother said.

"Yes, do," said the aunt, smiling. "Are we in it?"

One writes what one cannot say, I thought.

After we had gobbled up finger sandwiches, petits fours, and sipped our teacups dry, the others began haggling over the bill. I turned to Camille, a fellow writer whose sensitive, practical nature I admired. Although I knew I was treading on dangerous ground by bringing up the subject again, I couldn't resist. I wanted her advice about writing.

"Tell the truth," she said, without a pause. She didn't know the topic, only that its subject was "difficult and intense."

Tell the truth.

One truth was that Henry—who had come to my rescue, who had never doubted my story or judged me, who had honored my need for a "grace period" after the rape, agreeing to avoid physical intimacy for fear of causing in me a "bad reaction"—was now *her* boyfriend. He sat nearby, mostly bald, looking frightfully middle-aged.

Had he ever told her about the rape, I wondered? Certainly it was not something *we* had since talked about.

Camille regarded me through her eyeglasses, half-smiling. We all know secrets about each other, even when we think we don't. We sense the weak spots.

Weeks later, when I was packing, I came across

the manuscript of my stream-of-consciousness poem, "a hurried lullaby," tucked inside a folder of Simon's letters to me and other related documents. I couldn't read the words then. Just seeing the folder always gave me chills. In my seven-page account of the incident, which, ironically, was typed on the back of blank itinerary forms, I had purposely described what had happened in a clinical way, recording only the facts. Otherwise, I was afraid that my memory of that experience might contort the truth, sinking so deep into my subconscious as to be unrecognizable. Aside from numbness, I wasn't aware of what I felt anyway. The pages were paper-clipped together, along with a fortune: "Friends will always rush to your defense at the slightest occasion."

I thought of Henry's voice on the phone: *Sure, I can help.* What if the incident in Hawaii hadn't happened? Would Henry and I still be together? One never knows. Somewhere a butterfly's lifted wings are frozen.

I touched the pages tentatively and peered inside each envelope, aware of the power these artifacts still had over me. There were also three unsent postcards: "Bird's Eye View of Waikiki and Diamond Head," "Makapuu Beach," and "Waikiki Beach in the Moonlight." I stared at the postcards for a long time, and then added everything to my suitcase. I felt like Pandora, tempting wrath with my curiosity. But it needed to be done.

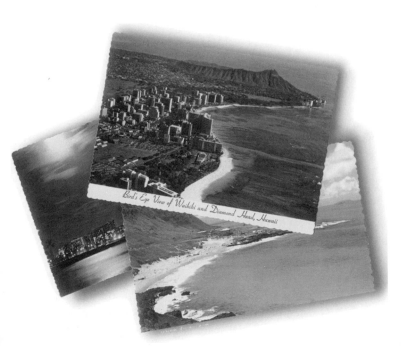

Bird's Eye View of Waikiki and Diamond Head, Hawaii

Labyrinth

The last days of the millennium were peculiar and stressful. I was consumed by the holidays, the logistics of my trip to London, and a plethora of domestic tasks, all of which needed doing in a short span of time. Racing from place to place, I checked things off my list, only to add another two. Apparently I was not alone in my chaotic feeling, for I noticed a quiet searching look in many people's eyes. The lady at the Post Office, spooked by the digital countdown blinking on the wall behind her, confided to me her worries about the apocalypse.

I had watched the fireworks on TV when the millennium officially dawned in Aukland, New Zealand. Now it was passing like a shooting star across the globe, toward San Francisco where I was. Shying away from the revelry, I decided that I would honor the occasion by walking the labyrinth at Grace Cathedral. Designed after the medieval one in Chartres, France, it had drawn me to its center many times.

Labyrinth

There was a certain mystery about this labyrinth; I had often experienced a subtle shift of consciousness when I dared step inside its circuitous path. I usually walked it on my birthday or when I was confused, uncertain, and had a question to ask. Rounding the twists and turns, clearing my mind and heart as I went, I was always led to a place where, in the balm of silence, consoled and uplifted by the colorful stained glass windows, I discovered, once again, that I had been on the path all along.

Perhaps I was open to this because of my early childhood experiences creating stone circles in the backyard and the joy I felt performing the May Pole Dance. Or maybe it was just the bubble of time for reflection and intuition seductively offered in that sacred space. All I knew was that from my first encounter with the labyrinth, something resonated, and I felt a strong, if curious, affinity.

I didn't know, of course, that like a wise, old friend, the labyrinth had appeared in my life just when I needed it most. I was simply open to it as a spiritual tool and respected its gifts of insights and guidance.

Although Nob Hill was bustling with partygoers that night, Grace Cathedral stood aloof. Its grand, white steps and moonlit steeple looked inviting. I passed through the heavy doors, entering a world lit by flickering white candles and dwarfed by the bold and passionate organ music. There was a breathless feeling inside the cathedral.

I removed my shoes and waited for the knot of people at the labyrinth's entrance to disperse. With less than an hour left to make my way along the path, I closed my eyes and marveled at where I had been, wondering what I would make of the rest of my life and giving thanks

111

that I was still here. I could have been a statistic. The subject of a sad article in the local paper. A fine-printed obituary.

Studying the labyrinth's dizzy purple pattern, I felt overwhelmed. Yet a labyrinth, unlike a maze, has no intention to baffle or mislead. It is unicursal, meaning that one path leads both in and out without dead-ends or tricks. I knew that I might side-step a path and find myself suddenly going in the wrong direction, but I couldn't get lost, at least, not physically so. Still, I hesitated.

I ought to mention here a little about the unusual history of labyrinths. Born of nature's spiral—think fingerprints, tide pools, and sunflowers, all of which form a curving, convoluted path reaching simultaneously inward and outward—they appear throughout the world in different cultures and religions as an icon of humanity. A mystical tool, labyrinths have been used for ritual dancing, healing, pilgrimage, as a link to the afterlife, and as a source of grace. Prehistoric aboriginal labyrinths were meant "to guide future initiates in their mental processes." Indigenous African, Indian, and Chinese, among other peoples, all call upon the spiral pattern when in need of purification and/or protection. Native Americans use its design in therapeutic sand paintings. Pagans believe that spirits dwell in the labyrinth's center.

In Greek mythology, the Minotaur is a monster, half man, half bull. On the king's command, a labyrinth was built in the palace of Knossos, which served as the Minotaur's prison. There the Minotaur was fed a diet of sacrificial Athenian young men and maidens. No one who had ever entered the labyrinth had been known to return.

Aiming to save future prey, heroic Theseus volunteered, offering himself as a victim. As he made his way in, he unwound a ball of golden thread given to him by the king's daughter, Ariadne, who had fallen in love with him. After slaying the Minotaur, he was able to escape by following the thread back out to her.[5]

For Christians, the permeation of the labyrinth and subsequent return to the world symbolizes spiritual death and rebirth. In medieval times, it mirrored the pilgrim's path to the holy land via the stations of the cross and from a state of sin to one of salvation.

Following the footsteps of pilgrims and mystics and brave Theseus before me, I stepped inside. It was the last time I would have this experience in the 20th century. I became aware of the others walking the labyrinth with me, imagining them as wispy spirits contained within bodies. Nearby people were singing and chanting while sitting on crowded pews. I wished that I could stop time and preserve this experience. At times I wanted to cry, but didn't. Instead I kept my head bowed, watching the path.

At one point, I thought of a poem by Rumi, the 13th-century Persian mystic who inspired the Sufi sect of whirling dervishes.

> *Keep walking, though there's no place to get to.*
> *Don't try to see through the distances.*
> *That's not for human beings. Move within,*
> *but don't move the way fear makes you move.*

Was I moving with fear, I wondered? Would some part of me always be carrying the rape's burden?

Treading lightly in the mutable realm of the present moment, I had no agenda for this walk. It was enough, on the millennium's eve, to simply let the path lead me. Pacing this way and that, sometimes pausing, my emotions fluctuating with each footfall, I made an unexpected turn and reached the labyrinth's center.

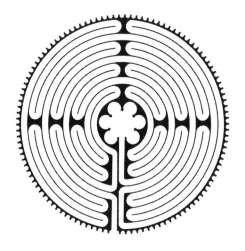

Instinctively I knelt down, closed my eyes, and meditated, recoiling into myself, teetering there, aware of my essence. I don't know how long I stayed in this position. Others must have joined me in the center, perhaps sitting or standing on one of the rosette's other petals, but I wasn't aware of them. It was a pure and golden time, without distraction. Only as a distant, separate reality did I notice any other activity in the church—the chalice of wine, the broken bread, the slowly murmured recitations. I was more taken by the frozen moment now melting within me, invisible tears waiting to fall.

Finally I stood and looked above me at the cavernous, vaulted ceiling. How small I felt! I bowed to the labyrinth's center, honoring in that simple gesture all the pain and magic of the past and my fear and excitement about the way the world might be tomorrow. Then I exited the same way I had come in. Around and around I went, lost in a swirl of people, light, and sound.

It was nearing midnight; soon the tower bells would ring, and we would gather in the foyer to sing "Auld Lang Syne." I was slowly meandering out, a feeling of gratefulness in my heart, when suddenly I heard these words within me, as though announced through an angelic megaphone: *You left some ghosts in this labyrinth at Grace Cathedral.* Ghosts? I knew exactly what was meant. I stopped right there on the path, temporarily blocking the other pilgrims, as I scribbled the message onto a scrap of paper.

Looking back, I saw the two evil ones depart, sulking away with their knife. I drew in a breath. For the first time in a long, long time, I was alone. I felt lighter.

---

[5]Curiously, around the time of the rape, like the labyrinth's architect, Daedalus himself, Henry began constructing an elaborate maze of cardboard and Elmer's glue. It remains unfinished.

Part III

It just simply divided my life, cut across it like that. So that everything before that was just getting ready, and after that I was in some strange way altered, ready. It took me a long time to go out and live in the world again. I was really 'alienated,' in the pure sense. It was, I think, the fact that I really had participated in death, that I knew what death was, and had almost experienced it. I had what the Christians call the 'beatific vision,' and the Greeks called the 'happy day,' the happy vision just before death. Now if you have had that, and survived it, come back from it, you are no longer like other people, and there's no use deceiving yourself that you are. But you see, I did: I made the mistake of thinking I was quite like anybody else, of trying to live like other people. It took me a long time to realize that that simply wasn't true, that I had my own needs and that I had to live like me.

KATHERINE ANNE PORTER
American short story writer, on surviving
the influenza plague at the end of World War I.

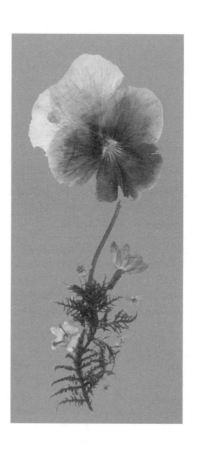

Safe Passage

On the same day I left San Francisco, a letter was posted to me from St. James's Church, Piccadilly, London, asking about my involvement with labyrinths. Although I had been corresponding sporadically with its sender over the last few years, I couldn't help but notice the synchronicity. Something was up. In fact, this was only the beginning of a thread of synchronistic events and encounters. In the labyrinth of my life, I was taking another small step forward.

Armed with notes and pen and laptop computer, I felt open to my task, yet also a shade apprehensive. The challenge of writing seemed less like choice, more like necessity and perhaps compulsion. The memory itself demanded its own liberation. I wondered how long it would take to reach a place of healing. After years of residual fear, the concept of inner ease seemed foreign to me. How did untraumatized people feel? Were the ghosts really that far behind me?

The airplane ascended through soft layers of clouds

then glided into an infinity of blue. *Angel territory*, I thought, gazing down at the distant changing landscape of desert and mountain, of winding pathways of water. I was between worlds. I was on my way.

I had finally uprooted myself from my unhappy home life in San Francisco. Amazingly, I had recreated a situation there that mirrored my feelings during the incident in Hawaii. The man with whom I had lived for many years, though lovable and supportive, was prone to intimidating rages. (This he blamed on being Italian.) When upset, he would stomp about and shout at me with operatic fury, which triggered my fears. Not only that, our belligerent "neighbor from Hell," whose throbbing music penetrated the thin bedroom wall behind my desk, caused me to feel invaded, even while in my own home. Pressure was building, but it seemed there was nowhere to retreat. By allowing these elements of my past—feeling unsafe, violated, trapped—to repeat themselves, I was unwittingly providing myself with another opportunity to heal. If only I had known that then.

And so, at the invitation of a friend, I arrived in London, desperately in need of a sabbatical—and with a story to tell.

My host knew nothing of my writing plans, yet one of the first things he did was show me a parchment reproduction of a 1728 poster, which he had purchased while on holiday. He laughed as he read the words, as though decreeing them.

REWARD
of
£150
is offered by His Majesty's Government
for information leading
to the capture of two
HIGHWAYMEN
known to be causing grief among
Travellers in these Parts
by Robbery of great violence
Render this countryside free
from such fiendish rogues
and make safe passage for all Travellers

I tried to laugh along, if a bit half-heartedly. Then a friend of my host's stopped by. Enthusiastic and full of life, she was studying to be an art therapist. Without prompting, she told me about her friend who had recently been raped. As she spoke, I began to feel uneasy. Not only was I unable to respond to her story in an authentic way by acknowledging my own history, but the circumstances of her friend's experience were especially disturbing. Still, I shook my head and empathized as best I could.

After a party that night, as my host and I returned to the flat, we noticed that the area leading up to the front door was occupied by police. It seemed that they were bent over something—or someone? A uniformed man approached and sternly advised us, "walk 'round the other way, please, because there's blood on the sidewalk."

Lying in bed later, I listened to the erratic sound of a revving engine. Finally, with annoyance, I got up and

121

peeked out the window at searchlights sweeping up and down the nearby railroad tracks. Something wasn't right. The "Reward" poster, the raped woman, the blood, and now this all conspired to produce in me an anxiety attack. While I struggled to think rationally (*it's not a manhunt, they're probably just working on the tracks, that's all*), old memories circled back. Even the black, reflective window with its homely British drapes reminded me of those billowing orange curtains in the tropics which had offered me an elusive form of peace as I lay there trembling.

When in a dangerous situation, people typically fight or flee (the fight/flight response) or they become immobilized. Yet it never occurred to me to jump out that window. It was too high up, and the prospect of landing on the cement courtyard, if I'd made it that far, wouldn't have had much appeal, even if I had been buffeted by the wisteria. Since fighting those two wasn't a possibility, I had frozen instead in numb submission.

But that's not happening *now*, I told myself.

The Scream

The London sky is shrouded in a pinkish-white haze. As I write, *Moonlight Sonata* plays on the radio. It is such a darkly rich and truthful piece of music. I used to play it on the piano, just barely getting the notes and timing right. It is the sort of song that weights memory, pulls it down under like a great anchor plunging to the bottom of the sea. Yet something isn't right, for in the rhythmic sway of seaweed, the rocking of water, the arm raised in slow motion, the knife, there is no scream. That one shrill penetrating siren-scream is somewhere inside of me, still waiting to come forth.

I feel like that terrified soul in "The Scream," the painting by Munch. While its trauma manifested in a hideous expression surrounded by swirls of color, mine is more subtle. As time passed, and my response to violence remained internalized, the alarm within me didn't dissipate but became instead an even greater psychic burden.

Words help. One by one, they lead me to a place

123

of acceptance and understanding. They form a bridge between worlds, helping me to honor the embryonic scream in its stillborn state.

How would the scream sound, were I to open my mouth now? It would be worse than a banshee's mournful wail, for it would express, not another's, but rather my own impending death. It would be full of fear and rage and sorrow. Windows would shatter. It would cause birds everywhere to suddenly take flight, filling the sky with an omen of restless wings.

Yet even before I can take a breath, my scream is always stopped, its tumultuous aria withheld. There is nothing more powerful than a woman's scream. The world does not want to hear it.

As testament to the synchronicity that has governed my life, Rimsky-Korsokoff's mischievous and sadly passionate *Scheherazade Suite* plays now on the radio. Like her, I want and need to tell my story. My scream may be mute, but the bowl of my silence is overflowing.

Keeper of Memory

The body knows, and carries within it, a visceral language of memories. While the ancient Egyptians believed that all thoughts and feelings began in the human heart and that it, rather than the brain, was the keeper of memories, according to psychiatrist and mystic C.G. Jung—.

Alas, while writing the above, I lost a paragraph in the computer. I was trying to copy and move it, but failed. Disillusioned, and provoked by the irony that I can't remember the important point I was about to make about memory, I leave the flat and stop by a nearby patisserie. "Nothing's ever lost. You just have to find a way to retrieve it," says a man there, when he overhears my story. "Use your intuition."

I come back and try. It's too late for the "undo" button, so I go to "start," like he'd said, and fiddle around in "settings" and "programs." In Microsoft Word, I search for help, cursing that little animated paperclip known as the Office Assistant, who, by his irritating range of facial expressions, provides no help at all and only seems to mock my efforts. I check the recycle bin, but it's empty. No matter what I do, nothing works. The writing is gone.

And then it dawns on me: Just as this information is inaccessible while mysteriously lodged somewhere in the brain of my computer, so too is a fragment of memory from that night in Hawaii still within me—specifically, when Hyena returned alone and raped me. I see him standing before me now, in frozen silhouette, moving neither forward or back, but that is all. It is as though time is a vacuum. There are no sensations—no foreboding sound of shoes on the floor, no awareness of a blade, no noxious smell of cigarettes—on which to hook a thought. I have only him— always there, never arriving, and therefore never departing. It is unfinished. I feel nothing.

Knowing that the memory exists somewhere is, and is not, a comfort. Despite its obscure invisibility and corresponding gap of feeling, it nevertheless persists and continues to affect me. How, I wonder, and in what ways? It is hard to conquer such a memory when it remains hidden.

Knot Spell

Returning to these memories is like reconstructing a magical (and therefore dangerous) tapestry which, from neglect, had dissolved into a pool of colored threads. Nevertheless, I must dip my hands in and work thread by thread to restore it. It is a frustrating and treacherous task, because the threads tangle and it seems that the more I am determined to sort them out, the worse my hands are marked by their indelible colors.

Blood-red and aquamarine weave with gold and white, green and black. A pattern begins to emerge, and I see that it contains me. The image is of a woman bound by serpentine coils of fear and mistrust, her spirit betrayed.

It is always alarming to see what one has become, though worse not to dare in the first place that possible disappointment. Still, healing can only occur with an awareness of where one is, here and now. It is useless trying to dismiss truth.

The background of menacing palm trees, moonlit

water, and Escher-like stairs leading nowhere intensifies. The woman's garment—a thin blue nightgown—radiates sadness. Yet it is the same color as the infinite sky and the pearly sea.

As I continue to work, I think of ancient Egyptian knot spells, those carefully and deliberately tied patterns which, by their voodoo-like influence, brought certain good or bad consequences.

With each pull of thread, there is the sense of a puzzle completed. Each stitch is exactly where it should be and relates in a small though perfect way to the next. Where before there were gaps and confusion, now there is growing order. As I stop to look at my work, the scene becomes clearer and, paradoxically, loses some of its power.

Naming the Unnamable

This morning, I am trying to decide on fictional names for the two rapists. It is Sunday, a day when most other people in London are probably relaxing or attending church.

Their real names were not known to me at the time of the incident, so using them would give a slanted view, making monsters seem more human. Although I am aware of their ethnic backgrounds (Dutch and Portuguese) it would be inappropriate to refer to them as such. Also, I suppose I am trying to protect myself, for fear of retribution. Yet I must call them something, even if I resent the effort required. Up to this point, I have been using scribbled Xs to refer to them, but now more is needed. I feel alternately sad and lightheaded as I pore over books about mythological creatures, trying to find a match. I want to show how they appeared as nameless entities to me, acquiring identities only by virtue of their deeds and actions.

While the tall man resembled a cavalier giraffe

when I first encountered him with Simon, only then did he behave in the manner of that animal. Later that night, he became more of a hyena.

The ancient Arabs believed that if a hyena crossed a man's shadow, the man would be unable to speak or move. Bartholomew, a 16th-century writer, claimed that an animal would be charmed into a state of immobility if a hyena circled it three times. I had a similar reaction, for my encounter with him resulted in what can only be described as a "paralysis of spirit" from which I am still trying to free myself.

No one likes hyenas. There is something menacing about them. They are hunters and scavengers, motivated by the scent of blood. Their wild, uncontrollable whoop is said to resemble a human laugh, giving them the nickname, "laughing hyena." But it is not really laughter, rather something more eerie and malicious.

Is Simon home? Ha ha ha. We're friends of his.

Hyenas intimidate as they prowl the night. Due to their bone-crushing jaws, other animals—be they large or small—shiver in their presence. The hyena is unstoppable; in his desire for meat, he will be led to innocence.

While this name comes easily, the other's doesn't.

Even at the time, I sensed that while Hyena lacked a conscience, the other man possessed one, though clearly it was lost, displaced, or ignored that night. The tragedy for him, I believe, is that he will always have that memory of his disgrace.

Anything could have happened; they could easily have killed me. Yet I instinctively interpreted their individual capacity for violence in different ways. Hyena was a carnivore. He did whatever needed to be done to sustain himself. Pleasure was taken as a byproduct of violence. The other passed through my nightmare in a different way.

I slowly turn the pages of a book. Bear, no. I like bears. Boar, bull, dragon, lion, lizard, owl, pig, serpent, and wolf are all possibilities, but none seems right. I remember him as stealthy, like a raccoon, with the fierceness of a panther, and of course there was an ominous quality about him too, like a raven—though in truth he seemed neither human nor animal, but rather phantomlike.

Turning to a section on the Egyptians, I find the name Seth. This was the god of evil and darkness. Seth is shown as a man bearing the head of an unidentifiable creature, whose snout, pricked ears, and tail are reminiscent of a dog's. I try the name Seth. Wrong.

Hours pass. The faint blue sky darkens with clouds. I am losing a day to this pursuit.

I think of Native American names which tell so much in their simplicity. Names like Two Whistles and Trickster. I see him bent over me, like a cloud blocking all light.

And then I know. *Dark One.*

Sorry Traveler

Again I ask myself: *What if I had never boarded that plane, if I had stayed home, if I had never written to Simon again... Could I have avoided trauma? Or would it have found me somewhere else?* These are unanswerable questions, the same sort of "wild regrets," about which Oscar Wilde wrote. Like Zen koans, they have the tendency to expand mystery rather than reducing it.

And so I am left with uncertainties, while secretly wishing for a better past. I try to train myself to focus on the "what is" rather than the "what ifs." I often fail.

Goethe said that, "As long as you do not know how to die and come to life again, you are but a sorry traveler on this dark earth." And perhaps I am like that, making my way along life's labyrinthine passages, feeling afraid. Or, if not afraid, then mad and bitter. Cheated. After all, I was only twenty.

This broken moment follows my joy like a hound, I wrote in a poem.

At my core, I *know*. I know that I have been somewhere, seen something. I suppose my nightmarish instruction—that each moment *is* eternity's gift—is not unlike the exhilaration thrill seekers experience when they plunge off bridges, attached only by their umbilical-like bungee cords. If only I could remember it.

But tonight, like the spirits of the dead in Greek mythology, I wish that I could drown my sorrows by drinking from Lethe, the river of forgetfulness.

Lucky

Highgate Cemetery, London. It is a gorgeous day. In the nearby park, children are rolling down soggy hills, yet I feel anxious. I walk past the tombstones in a hurry.

Lime green moss covers some of the graves. Daffodils and primroses sprout from others. Stone angels with bowed heads and broken fingers and hands guard the dead. The tips of their wings snag the late afternoon light. Everything is still, but the randomly squawking crows and whirring wasps. Domino, the black-and-white cemetery cat, is somewhere hiding.

Karl Marx is buried here. And many lesser-known souls, whose names speak in soft, sepulchral murmurs from the carved headstones.

When the hand-bell is rung, signaling closing time, I pause before the grave of John Pitt Kennedy, who died in November of 1897. I picture a frumpish man with a handlebar moustache. Seeing his name, Kennedy, and the date he died reminds me of my birthday, in November

Lucky

1963. I was home sick from school, and my mother and I had turned on the television to pass the time. We watched John F. Kennedy riding down the Dallas street in his open car. Waving. And then, all at once, everything changed. The president was shot.

My education about such matters as fate and mortality had begun long before that. Looking back, I must have been a dreary child. I remember shuffling through the tall grasses of the field across from my family home, reciting a saying I had just heard: "You can't take it with you." Such a revelation—that material objects, especially money, meant nothing in the other realm. So what mattered? Apparently not the fifty-odd dollars I had squirreled away inside my small black safe. Only the pause following my question alluded to any suitable answer, for it represented Mystery, the greater unknown. That it was, by definition, hidden and withheld only made my interest keener. Yet I knew it existed; it was in the dome of sky and in the field all around me—I sensed it.

Recently I read that Madame Blavatsky whispered to herself as a child, apparently prompted by some inner communion. I never whispered to myself, preferring to observe and listen. Eventually I came to realize that, whatever this Mystery was, it was large enough to embrace all the goodness of this world, as well as any evil inherent in it. For without one half of truth, the other is incomplete, out of balance, misrepresented. The moon needs the dark sky in which to rise.

I gaze at the shadowed path, absorbing the abundant silence. Sighing in the sultry air, I continue on, treading in the footsteps of mourners.

Once my mother and I were driving home together from The Barn, a large red structure that housed many small international restaurants under one roof. I was in the back seat, gnawing on a semi-transparent chunk of rock candy that resembled quartz crystal. As dusk turned to night, the brooding clouds overhead erupted into explosive rainshowers. I watched my mother grip the Buick's steering wheel. Like a number of women of that time, she was uncertain of her driving skill. Cursing, she set the windshield wipers into fast motion. Still sucking my rock candy, I became hypnotized by their frantic, futile rhythm. I could taste disaster. There was nothing to see but the rain's rippling silk, which, whipped aside by the wipers, revealed yet more rain, and beyond that, a dense and stubborn fog. "I can't see where I'm going!" she cried, panicked. We inched along the narrow winding road as slowly as was possible, without actually stopping. Only a miracle—God's hand parting the sky—could change the weather; it was all up to her. The challenge of the blurry road, punctuated by the rain's erratic stammer, created a drama in which we were the leading characters, and the rest of the world, if not the entire universe, conspired as villain. I realized that we would not know the outcome of this story until it had been lived through. Although the precise variety of struggle was new, the plot itself, in which my mother was both victim and heroine, seemed not unfamiliar to her. I could tell, by the way her face had gone slack, that she was calling on all her accumulated wit and intelligence—her survival skills—to navigate us back home.

Afterwards, parked in the driveway, she sat in the

car for a moment, angry, upset, electrified, and muttering with relief, *We were lucky.*

I suppose we were. Because apparently bad things happened. Nothing was guaranteed. My education as her daughter included the ability to recognize calamities large and small, and the tenacious gypsy spirit to overcome them. "It's a great life if you don't weaken," she often said. Heaven itself took on a dodgy, rustic quality whenever she referred to it as "The Great Beyond."

Later, in my room, when I was tucked safely in bed, I might have had my recurring nightmare about the witch who lived in the field across from our house. That same field, which filled with amber poppies during summer, was where I had run from my father, talked to Simon among the oaks, and where I had had the childhood revelation about materialism and death. When ponds formed, it was there I caught those primeval beings known as polliwogs. Sometimes I walked across the field to visit the nuns' convent, which, like an elusive mirage, always had a way of staying just far enough from me as to be unreachable. It was in that field, too, that I had "lost" my virginity.

Places have always taught me. They offer up the sort of information meant for poets, in the way the breeze skirted past, carrying with it the scent of eucalyptus and acacia trees. Or by the sinister sound of shushing tide. Sometimes this information was accessible, other times not. I had to be open, to look and listen for it.

Now, in Highgate Cemetery, at closing time, I glance at the hunched black crows dotting distant branches. A British man strolls past. "Do not ask for whom the bell tolls!" he proclaims, a bit too cheerfully.

Listening to the watery sound of the clanging bell, I feel soothed and then unsafe in the silence that follows. For I know that, sooner or later, it will toll for me.

The Empty Mirror

"Only two things are certain in this world: that we are born alone and that we die alone," Richard Leven, RAF pilot, circus ringmaster, palmist, and a late friend of mine used to say. Richard had survived numerous near-misses during World War II as he flew sorties over Europe, witnessing the loss of life of nearly everyone around him while he remained miraculously untouched. It is no wonder that after the war was over, he found circus life so intriguing (that fantasy world of tigers, elephants, and horseback-riding ballerinas somehow balanced the horrors of falling bombs and concentration camps). His war-time experiences left him with a bittersweet nature and the gift of second-sight.

A brush with death can result in an impossible mix of feelings: Relief. Gratitude. Shock. Sorrow. Anger. Guilt. It can also instill in one a profound and startling awareness.

Death beckoned to me that night in Hawaii, filling

the room with its greedy presence. The bedroom window, shrouded in amber curtains, became a portal to an alternate reality somewhere beyond the empty moonlit street, the stormy galaxies, an unknown void into which I might uneasily slip.

Considering that death promised nothing, yet wanted everything from me, its pull, like a magnetic lure, was great—similar to that overwhelming desire one has to jump when leaning over a rooftop railing. It waited nearby, expectantly, with the force of a whirlpool. Apparently death is always here; it feeds on time. Strange that it had managed to stay so well-hidden before this.

The bed on which I lay had but one purpose: to offer my body as sacrifice. I wonder now about that bed's history. Who had slept in it before me? And who is sleeping in that same spot by the window now? It is conceivable that children have jumped up and down and laughed there. Or perhaps a knot of disharmonious energy remains, creating arguments between lovers, causing unsettling chills and shudders.

That night, death was generous. I was given the chance to further appreciate this strange wonderland and myself in it. The two men may have robbed me of nearly everything else, but death left behind a calling card with its name written in ash as a sad souvenir of its visit.

Yet that night was also my rebirth, for I was forced awake, made to witness this life, to fully inhabit the moment. There is no doubt that it produced in me an altered state. Even as the situation devolved into cruelty, there was within it a curious seed of goodness. Violence can be grace's unlikely catalyst.

Although I felt emotionally anesthetized for years after the attack, my sense of compassion was silently building. The saying, "If not for the grace of God go I," took on less abstract meaning. For I had learned that there was nothing protecting me from the whims of fate but my own haphazard prayers and the occasional intervening angel.

When death comes again and if I sense that it is inevitable, I will try to be more welcoming. It's the only way to be when confronted by an empty mirror, which, in contrast to one's dying self, seems oddly rich and abundant. Death is a trickster. In its own awkward way it tries to bring peace, to comfort. It knows that a state of nothingness is far more desirable than a glimpse of that which is already lost.

Of course, one can try to turn back. "Sorry, another time, perhaps..." Yet even that, if granted, is only a temporary solution. As much as we would like to think otherwise, death is a certainty. Richard was right.

Wrong Time, Wrong Place

Maybe I deserved it, I think. It is the sort of rationale to which health professionals, like Dr. O., object. "It's not your fault," they say. "You're not responsible."

Of course not. How could I be? Still, there's always a small, nagging voice inside, asking, *But what if I am?*

I was brought up in a quasi-Christian environment, which acknowledges sin and resurrection (the body born again after death) but not karma and reincarnation (the soul reborn into a different body) and am curious to reconcile the two.

Karma (Sanskrit for "action" or "work") is the moral law of cause and effect. According to the Hindu mystical writings known as the Vedas, it governs our lives (including previous lives and any future ones), rewarding or punishing our behavior by propelling us into situations of sickness or health, riches or poverty. A concept such as this can be provocative, for it implies that we are responsible for the bad things that happen to us, therefore robbing us of our victimhood. In other words, there are no accidents.

Some see karma as a "subtle type of matter that attaches itself to the soul." *Ahimsa*, the principle of respect for and practice of non-injury to all living things, is based on the idea that those who commit violent acts, whether great or small, are harmed themselves. This is the justice that I imagine has colored the lives of Hyena and Dark One. What more suitable punishment could there be for such a man than to be sentenced to live within the prison of himself?

Perhaps karma is nothing more (or less) than the cumulative effect of all one's thoughts, deeds, and actions, and those of one's ancestors too.[1] Virginia Woolf addressed this poetically when she wrote about her sexual molestation by her half-brother, Gerald Duckworth, "It proves that [I] was not born on the 25th January 1882, but was born many thousands of years ago; and had from the very first to encounter instincts already acquired by thousands of ancestresses in the past."

In my own history, the ancestors on my father's side are Scottish. These people are known for their dour manner (blame it on the icy wind), a dance called the Highland Fling, and their legendary thriftiness. The Scots also have a bloody history of murdering each other. In their sleep. With daggers, swords, and knives. Perhaps I was once on the blade's other side.

Although it makes sense to me that there must be a "recycling" of ourselves, if only as the redistribution of our molecules in the universe (as well as some spiritual equivalent of this), I find it challenging to accept the idea that I will one day cease to exist in the form I now know.

The notion of karma hinges on an afterlife. Polynesians (from whom the first Hawaiians descended) believed that the afterlife was located on a faraway island, a mountain, or underground. The ancient Egyptians, who were strangely pragmatic about such things, provided food for the dead and mapped out the passage between realms in guidebooks (*The Book of Two Ways, The Book of Gates*). Because of the sudden demarcation imposed upon my psyche, *this* life, now, feels like my afterlife.

Was it my karma to be raped? Was some ancient wrong righted by my misfortune? (And was it my friend Martin's karma to be found lying shattered and unconscious by the side of the road? What possible benefit can come from that?) Or, was it simply the impersonal effect of "wrong time, wrong place"? I still don't know.

---

[1]Consider these words of W. Jerome Harrison's "Light as a Recording Agent of the Past," in *The Photographic News*, 1886: "It is a wonderful thought that every action which has ever occurred on this sun-lit earth of ours—or indeed, for that matter, anywhere within this illuminated universe—is recorded by the actions of light, and is at this moment visible somewhere in space, if any eye could be placed there to receive the waves of light....The very idea should stimulate us to do nothing that will not bear developing and exhibiting to the gaze of mankind."

Lightning Strikes

The London weather is unsettled. Spring has shown its face, only to be masked by a dreary, foreboding sky. Clouds usually dot the weather maps here—white, black, or white-and-black. Today, thundershowers are predicted.

What is evil? I wonder, as I ponder the gathering clouds. It is not easily defined. While some think it is a purely moral issue, its most commonly agreed-upon characteristic is that it causes pain—whether of a physical, emotional, and/or psychic nature. And whether God wills evil, merely allows it, or is powerless to prevent it remains a mystery. When I think of evil, I imagine those three monkeys with their hands covering eyes, ears, and mouth—*see no evil, hear no evil, speak no evil*—denying its existence by blinding, muting, and silencing themselves.

The mushroom cloud over Hiroshima has become a symbol of evil and human suffering,[2] which, though it is widely recognized, is still beyond most of our comprehension. Only when one comes face to face with the reality of evil as the victim of a crime or similar unfortunate event, can one really begin to understand it. Until such time, evil is only abstract.

Perhaps there are only evil acts, not evil people— acts that are unleashed through both willing and unwilling channels. It makes me think of lighting. Lightning, like the outworking of evil, can also cause severe damage. This fiery force imprinting the sky with its harsh, unruly brilliance, is the very signature of a demon. There are different types of lightning: red sprites, blue jets, and elves. Yet even such innocuous-sounding names do not change the fact that lightning, when it strikes, can suck the life-giving waters from a person, leaving them soul-shocked, if not completely dead. There is a certain absolute power and sense of inevitability about both lightning and evil.

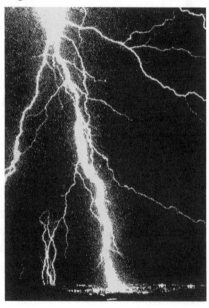

The negative charge created by a cloud produces a positive charge as it strikes the earth. Like yin and yang, good and evil are intricately linked. They co-exist. If evil is regarded as something other than us, apart from us, something we seek to root out but never understand or embrace, then evil will always follow us, striking as from a spring sky like a zigzagged bolt of lightning.

Oddly, the safest place to be during an electrical storm is out in the open, lying flat. What more vulnerable position could there be? And yet it is in that very position that lightning is least apt to find one. Alas, I suppose that is where the similarities stop, since that is how evil found me.

---

[2]So, too, since the writing of these words, have the nightmarish images of the World Trade Center.

Justice

The two men—whose names I had recorded in a blue scrawl and had then tried to forget about—have become for me representatives of evil. Yet I recognize that they are not evil; rather, evil had run through them. It had possessed and occupied them. Like a powerful ocean tide, they threatened my life, left their mark upon me, and then retreated. I wonder if they remember me, that faceless girl trembling on the bed, the one with whom they had been so intimate.

My compassionate self reminds me that someone who brings intense suffering to another must be suffering himself. Still, not everyone who is deeply hurting acts upon such feelings. And what about crimes committed in self-defense? Surely these acts can produce what is perceived as evil by its victim. How can such things be measured? After all, a crime is a crime is a crime—isn't it?

Surely a rapist would be considered an evil person, but taken in an objective light, what is he really but a tortured individual who has made a series of choices which have led him to act in a certain way and who must thereafter live with himself and his deeds? Although a man who rapes may not necessarily feel any remorse, I do believe that the act itself ultimately creates in the life of that person its own unique punishment.

I have always felt a strong aversion to the death sentence; it seems so obviously hypocritical to impose as punishment the very same crime that one is saying is wrong. I accept prison as a "necessary" evil[3] but only if, by transforming its inhabitants, it ultimately protects the innocent; otherwise it is no more than a breeding ground for further evil. Thomas Merton, Trappist monk and poet, wrote in *No Man is an Island:*

Compassion teaches me that my brother and I are one. That if I love my brother, then my love benefits my own life as well, and if I hate my brother and seek to destroy him, I destroy myself also. The desire to kill is like the desire to attack another with an ingot of red hot iron: I have to pick up the incandescent metal and burn my own hand while burning the other.

The notion of trying to control evil by imprisoning it reminds me of that old *I Love Lucy* skit in which Lucy and Ethel are working in a chocolate factory, trying to keep up with the constantly moving stream of chocolates on the assembly line. Their efforts are both ludicrous and futile.

"In the last resort there is no good that cannot produce evil and no evil that cannot produce good," wrote

Jung. The Holocaust, as well as other horrific historic events, consequently inspired a profound sense of compassion and appreciation of life. Even so, this is hardly any justification for evil, and probably no or little comfort for a survivor.

Pacifists endorse turning the other cheek. As Gary Zukav wrote:

> Non-judgmental justice is a perception that allows you to see everything in life, but does not engage your negative emotions. Non-judgmental justice relieves you of the self-appointed job of judge and jury because you know that everything is being seen—nothing escapes the law of karma—and this brings forth understanding and compassion. Non-judgmental justice is the freedom of seeing what you see and experiencing what you experience without responding negatively. It allows you to experience directly the unobstructed flow of the intelligence, radiance, and love of the Universe of which our physical reality is a part. Non-judgmental justice flows naturally from understanding the soul and how it evolves.

I find it difficult to be so enlightened when I look back at my last quarter century and realize that that one night has imposed itself upon every moment that has followed, tainting my youth with its bitter, soul-making medicine.

Still, the rape was a crucible, serving me, over time, by its alchemy of opposites, my "good" blending and fusing with their "evil" which, after nearly destroying me, created within me a renaissance of spirit. Although much was lost, I am today stronger and deeper as a human being because of it.

Such an initiation can work two ways. Perhaps, by their encounter with innocence, by feeling its stark opposite to the violence in their own veins, those two have learned something as well. Or perhaps not.

---

[3]In *Autobiography of a Yogi*, Paramahansa Yogananda is visited by his late guru, Sri Yukteswar, who reports on a unique form of prison in the afterlife: "Various spheric mansions or vibratory regions are provided for good and evil spirits. Good ones can travel freely, but the evil spirits are confined to limited zones."

Minotaur

What happened in Hawaii was one of my most significant, life-altering experiences, though I had rarely talked about it in all those intervening years. Imagine someone surviving any other type of calamity and keeping silent. It seems not only tragic, but also absurd.

Why, I had to ask myself, did I feel so ashamed? Especially after danger had passed, why did I feel it necessary to protect those two, to shield *their* story? There was no obvious answer to this. Other than the stigma associated with rape, I had nothing to hide. I had only woken up to the blade. Was that my fault? This caused me to think about others (mostly women and girls, though some men and boys) who feel the same. What cultural shame are we thus perpetuating by remaining silent? By doing so, we only further victimize ourselves. No one heals. And so the tragic dance continues.

I realize that in the very center of myself a monster still resides; he is my Minotaur. He may never go away. I picture him as twin-horned and with large cumbersome feet. He has the skin of an elephant and the eyes of a snake. His bay—a lone, lingering cry—is at once sad and terrifying. He is the keeper of all the frightful things of my life, the risks and terrors. I suppose we all have a Minotaur somewhere deep inside us. Taking Ariadne as guide, the trick is to learn how to slay him, not by sword, but with the greater weapon of love.

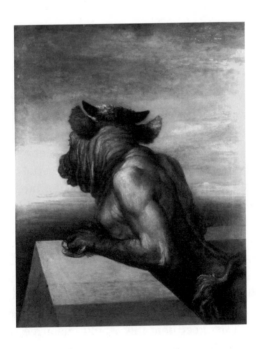

The Rape of the Locks

While it's true that the process of writing has been a positive experience, there have also been many moments of doubt, dread, and panic caused by the churning of this memory. I had not anticipated this. As Easter approached (and with it, the rape's anniversary), all the talk of Christ being nailed to the cross strongly affected me. I felt the nails. I *knew* that He had suffered. I thought of the curious connection between Christ and the scarab. Both are symbols of resurrection and rebirth, of darkness miraculously transformed into light.

Unfortunately, that didn't help. I slid into a depression. Not knowing what else to do, I decided to get my hair cut. Considering the ritual grooming practiced by primates, I assumed that this would cheer me up. I was wrong. My haircut resembled that of a Benedictine monk— no, a schoolgirl with a bowl turned over her head. Either way, it was precisely the opposite of what I'd asked for. For hours I played with the disaster, combing, mussing,

154

wetting down, then drying off. Nothing helped. I was distraught. No, distraught is not a strong enough word. Near-suicidal would be more accurate.

Worse than my appearance was the underlying feeling of having been *violated*. Whether this sense of violation was exacerbated by my personal history, I do not know. Yet as I trudged along the London streets in the rain, aware of my hideousness, I had a strange revelation: The anger, hurt, and disappointment which I feel as a result of the bad haircut seemed no less intense, in that moment, than what I felt about the rape. Their entwined roots ran extraordinarily deep.

I decided to get another haircut. This challenged my sense of trust by posing a risk: What if it turned out even worse than the one before it?

The new haircut, which I wear now as I write, is far from perfect. For one, it's too short and makes me feel like a sheared lamb. After years of long hair, my neck is cold. Still, it feels good to surrender vanity, to relinquish attachment.

Time heals all wounds. Hair grows.

Trespassed

After days of stormy weather, we now have powder-blue skies and sun. I open the window and lean outside. Spring is here! The ice cream van with its ice lollies, Carnival Cones, and Mister Magics passes cheerfully by, playing its tinkling song.

Some ants have wandered in and are now traversing my desk in search of food. "Retreat or perish!" I shout, shooing them away. There's something so innocent about ants. They meander along, oblivious to danger. I lure a few onto a postcard, so that I can nudge them back out onto the window ledge where they will be reunited with the others. I haven't the heart to actually harm them.

That done, it's back to work. I decide to consult the Oxford English Dictionary once again, this time for its definition of "forgive."

1. *to give, grant.*
2. *to give up, cease to harbour*

(resentment, wrath).
3. *to remit (a debt); to give up
   resentment or claim to acquittal
   for, pardon (an offense).*

That night, I was forced to give them what they wanted. Now I find that I don't want to give them anything else. I feel no high-minded benevolence toward them, no generous ease of spirit. And yet neither do I want to be the handmaiden of resentment—if only for my own good. I would rather be so strong that I am able to move from a place of feeling diminished to one of abundance.

For years the concept of forgiveness did not even occur to me. To forgive, one must first feel compassion. Perhaps I need to feel compassion for myself first, before I can offer it to them.

Across the column from "forgive" is the word "forget." "Pray you now, forget and forgive," said William Shakespeare.

While I want to cast away shame and purge myself of the rape's clinging shadow, I will never forget. Just as the flight of a butterfly affects the entire universe, so too has something been forever altered and changed inside of me. I am not the one who was before, but rather someone else. I am subtly damaged, and yet, by that very injury, shocked awake. Where did my dislodged soul go in those hours? To forget the trauma of that night would be to also ignore its gift.

Reciting the Lord's Prayer in that small white chapel as a young girl, I could never have suspected the significance that one line, *As we forgive those who have trespassed against us,* would have for me now. Nevertheless, the words resonated. At the time, the only trespass I knew was the childish prank of sneaking between rotting fence posts onto neighboring property, usually a sad and neglected-looking piece of land which, by its very desolation, invited what its owner sought to keep out. The trespasses alluded to in the prayer seemed to involve something far more significant and taboo.

When I think of forgiving those two, I feel numb. Although I try, I cannot freely disperse upon them any special blessing meant to free them (or myself) from some spiritual limbo. It doesn't seem my place to do this. Let God have that task.

Finding My Way

The path of healing can be indirect. Like the experience of traveling, it is not always so much about a destination, but rather the process by which one arrives. That is, *if* and *when* one arrives. I feel caught in the limbo of my uncertain quest. Still, the unhealed self demands transformation, whether by the manifestation of symptoms such as flashbacks and anxiety attacks or through a more general Nietzschean uneasiness which, once faced and tended to, can lead to positive change.

Faith is said to open the channel through which a Higher Power can intervene. This typically occurs either as a spontaneous "leap" of consciousness or is inspired by a faith healer. Whether the outcome of such faith is desired or not, I suppose it is still better to be like a flower and turn toward the light.

Dreams are useful healing tools, serving as compasses of the unconscious. The ancient Greeks practiced the ritual of incubation, passing the night in sacred spaces so that Asclepius, the god of medicine, could appear in their dreams with healing advice. In a recent dream of mine, I am walking in the field near where I grew up.

As I look back, water from a hose sprays me. It's Simon. Then we're in a theatre together; he is working there as a stagehand. Nearby there are seats filled with people. "Keep your distance," I tell him. He responds with humor. Then he shows me an antique postcard of Hawaii with palm trees. I say that I don't like it. He laughs. "We were there," he says, pointing to a corner of the postcard. "That's Honolulu..."

Simon appearing in this manner takes me by surprise. I feel betrayed by his presence. The hose is both phallic and a channel for water, which is symbolic of the divine. His use of the hose strikes me as foolish. Perhaps like a spirit who is trying to communicate with the living, it is the only way he knows how to make contact with me—by blasting me with a jolt of water from behind. It seems an oddly forceful act for a man whom I remember as mild and passive. Although next we are in a theatre, which suggests the unreal and perhaps even the absurd, I am aware of who he is in my life and have no tolerance for slippery meanings, even as a dreamer in a dream. My telling him to "keep his distance" is like raising a crucifix to deflect evil. Yet it doesn't seem to work. His humor startles and offends me; it feels not so much inappropriate as blind. He is behaving unconsciously—that is, until he shows me the postcard. This is what connects us. It also proves that it all happened—that there is someone else who remembers. The postcard serves as a mirror to my memories. It holds a reality within it, much like those plastic toy TVs that one angles up and down to shift the image. He is obviously aware of our past, though he doesn't take it seriously. I realize that he has moved on with his life, while I have not. I am left feeling that there is much misunderstood, and thus unresolved, between us.

A different dream:

I am in Hawaii, comparing it to how it is different than before. Mostly it has become more polluted and the buildings have decayed. There is lots of scaffolding all about, though not very many tourists. I am not afraid.

In this dream, I am wandering in a ghost town. It is as though I have been dropped down into this dense, greyish, mostly unpeopled environment by an unseen hand—returned to it not by my own will, but by another's. I am simply present, making observations with a sort of dislocated neutrality. Once, this place was beautiful and enchanting; now it is in disrepair, quietly ruined. Perhaps Hawaii is slowly dying in me?

I don't know what more these dreams of mine might mean, beyond what I have ventured above. I wonder what Asclepius would say, what advice, if any, he would give me.

Words have a unique energy. Indigenous peoples and clinical researchers have long recognized the therapeutic value of storytelling, which is not so much a learned art as a natural one. Shamans (who regard the cause of illness as "soul loss") channel the language of animals when they heal. This is similar to the Pentecostal

Church's divine healing practice of "speaking in tongues." Priestess Pythia also uttered seemingly incoherent words when she delivered the oracles at Delphi. I am aware of the charm of words, the way agony becomes art, as I write about Hawaii in these pages.

While it is hard to tell the truth, it is harder still to keep it in. Following a lifeline of words, I can return to that muggy night in Hawaii—stop time, examine, re-examine, go deeper—and feel in control of an uncontrollable event that had yet to occur. Writing gives me godlike powers.

Words have always been my saving grace. In the journals I've kept since I was twelve, all the ups and downs of my life are painstakingly recorded. Rarely, though, did I mention Hawaii (and ironically the dime store volume that might have shed light on that time was devoured by Vanessa's German shepherd). The stories I told in my fiction often related to the rape in some way, but, by not telling *my* story, I was, in a sense, denying what had really happened, therefore making it impossible to truly heal.

Still, I wrote every day. I wrote as though my life depended on it.

It did.

As I make this inward journey, I wonder if perhaps it is not a mistake that I feel I am going in circles on my healing path. For the circle symbolizes purity, unity, and wholeness of self; it is the labyrinth's essence. Many ancient peoples followed the labyrinth's meandering course around and around until they found themselves at its center. Mandalas, medicine wheels, and Sufi dervish dancing are all based upon this same primal pattern, which serves as an access to the realm of the divine. So maybe this circle of mine is leading me somewhere.

Will I ever be completely healed? I shy from the magic pills that are meant to ease the pain of PTSD but can also mask what may actually be a spiritual lesson in disguise. Talking therapy is another option, of course. I have already mentioned my failed forty-five minutes of therapy with Dr. O.

I carry on, that's all I can do. I put one foot in front of the other and pray that I will not encounter quicksand. The landscape ahead is of a mixed terrain, some parts craggy with ghostly trees, and yet, as I make my way past them, I see great, enchanted vistas up ahead.

Web Wisdom

My cousin is someone who lives by what she believes, seldom judging others and talking little about her faith—except in the context of the inspirational e-mails she regularly sends to me. I have always felt like the black sheep of the family—no husband, children, or mortgage. And yet, maybe because of the summers of bee stings and green apples we shared together as children, we are like sisters now; our differences of lifestyle seem to pose no threat to our bond. It's true that despite my dreamy nature, mine was always a more spontaneous existence. Even back then I was the one with the frown and torn dress, while she was sweet and demure and well-groomed. Only in the filigree bubbles of the bathtub did we become as equals, looking in a photo of that time like two old, giggling crones wearing hairnets.

After decades of letter writing, the transition to e-mail came easily, though I miss the dainty, scented floral paper that she used to write on. Still, for all our correspondence, I never told her about Hawaii. I guess I hesitated to ruin her innocent perception of me and of the world.

Once, when we were very young, I dreamt that she had hurt her hand. The next morning, after pressuring my mother to call her long distance, I discovered that she had. Blame it on Grandpa's sixth sense, working its ancestral charm. So I guess it isn't too surprising that while I am writing this book, her e-mails ("forwarded" from other sources) often correspond exactly with the very subject I am addressing—whether it is angels, the reasons bad things happen to good people, or just general paranoia (like her e-mail "Safety for Women" which offers useful tactics such as eye-gouging to avoid being the victim of a violent crime). Divine intervention is also a common theme.

Many of her e-mails revolve around trust in a Christian God and an acceptance of one's fate. Yet the stories of all religions share common threads. For example, "Things Aren't Always What They Seem," which derives from the Koran and tells of two traveling angels who stay in the homes of a rich couple and a poor couple, reminds me of the Taoist parable, "What is Bad, What is Good?" Here, an old farmer loses his best stallion. The next day, the stallion is returned to him, along with three wild mares. While riding one of the mares, the farmer's son falls and breaks his leg. Then an army official comes to the village, seeking men fit for war. The son is excused because of his broken leg. Each turn of the story causes neighbors to celebrate or bemoan the farmer's fate, while he alone remains wisely unswayed by circumstances.

Things aren't always what they seem. What is bad,

what is good?

One e-mail stands out from all the others by its touching, if chilling, quality.

Subject: Do What You Can

God has a way of allowing us to be in the right place at the right time. I was walking down a dimly lit street late one evening when I heard muffled screams coming from behind a clump of bushes.

Alarmed, I slowed down to listen and panicked when I realized that what I was hearing were the unmistakable sounds of a struggle: heavy grunting, frantic scuffling, and tearing of fabric.

Only yards from where I stood, a woman was being attacked. Should I get involved? I was frightened for my own safety and cursed myself for having suddenly decided to take a new route home that night. What if I became another statistic? Shouldn't I just run to the nearest phone and call the police?

Although it seemed an eternity, the deliberations in my head had taken only seconds, but already the cries were growing weaker. I knew I had to act fast. How could I walk away from this?

No, I finally resolved, I could not turn my back on the fate of this unknown woman, even if it meant risking my own life.

I am not a brave man, nor am I athletic. I don't know where I found the moral courage and physical strength—but once I had finally resolved to help the girl, I became strangely transformed.

I ran behind the bushes and pulled the assailant off the woman. Grappling, we fell to the ground, where we wrestled for a few minutes until the attacker jumped up and escaped.

Panting hard, I scrambled upright and approached the girl, who was crouched behind a tree, sobbing. In the darkness, I could barely see her outline, but I could certainly sense her trembling shock.

Not wanting to frighten her further, I at first spoke to her from a distance. "It's OK," I said soothingly. "The man ran away. You're safe now."

There was a long pause and then I heard the words, uttered in wonder, in amazement. "Dad, is that you?" And then, from behind the tree, stepped my youngest daughter, Katherine.

Do all the good you can, in all the ways you can, in all the places you can, at all the times you can, to all the people you can, as long as you ever can.

And some people say, "Don't get involved."

Faith

Ironically, I find myself working on this chapter at a time when I am lacking in faith and when what I need, more than anything else, is precisely that. Today I am hounded by a negative inner voice, lost in fear's circular thinking and hidden truths. I feel abandoned by the angels.

Faith is often a struggle for me. It is difficult for me to trust in the unfolding process of my life, to believe that despite outward circumstances, all is as it should be in any particular moment. And it is a hard to believe in the goodness of the world when it is, in fact, a violent place. Waking to find two men standing over my bed, glimpsing the knife, that sudden, bewildering, soul-wrenching constellation of pain has forever colored my perception. It was as though a trap door opened. Nothing could ever be taken for granted or counted on again.

After that, I felt rather like a visitor to earth, a bit ghostlike and unsettled in my ability to fit in and carry on as before. My self-importance, having been confronted with the possibility of its own obliteration, seemed to wilt rather than reassert itself. The survival of the actual rape was mostly automatic, the survival instinct being hard-wired in. It was during the aftermath, when shock subsided, that the world demanded that I adapt and establish with it a new relationship.

Whatever I had believed in before, however shallowly, had been simultaneously challenged and lost by what happened that night. A profound sense of vulnerability arises when one realizes that ultimately one has no control over the things that really matter. It is the motto of a victim, an anthem of helplessness, this soul-murdering uncertainty—but it is also fundamentally true.

Although I have moments when my faith soars, in common, everyday matters, I often falter. I don't blame myself; it's just that while others are storming confidently ahead, I am prone to feelings of doubt and dread. True faith, the kind that is continually renewed, reaffirmed, and reasserted, requires a gentle discipline. It is no use feeling smug, immune, or spiritually superior on this path. Everyone, no matter who she is, is constantly being tested.

My only consolation has been my rather intellectual understanding that there is a Higher Power guiding and informing us (should we choose to listen and obey) and at whose mercy we find ourselves daily. To think otherwise is worse than folly, for it implies that we are so special as to be somehow disengaged from the source that created and continues to provide for us. Behind our every action, whether outrageous or mundane, there is something greater, mysteriously propelling us.

I think of these words of Dylan Thomas:

The force that through the green fuse drives the flower
Drives my green age; that blasts the roots of trees
Is my destroyer.
And I am dumb to tell the crooked rose
My youth is bent by the same wintry fever.

Which is more powerful, I wonder, fear or faith? Fear has drawn me into its lair many times, sucking my vital spiritual blood from me. I would like to think that faith will win. It is not faith in a specific god or in any one dogma's dictates and promises, but faith as a natural, human response to what is perceived to be divine.

"Once I have decided, then this faith changes my position in the world, my attitude to the world; it establishes my fundamental trust and gives concrete shape to my trust in God." Faith, not fear, aligns us with the ways of nature, and dances us gracefully through life's changes. It creates possibilities. Fear dead ends; it obstructs and paralyzes.

Hoping to distract myself from my woes, I go to a party in Kensington where a gathering of literary types grazes in the twilit garden, clutching wine glasses. I wander about, dressed in lace and polka dots, trying my best to appear festive.

It works. A fair, pleasant woman approaches me right away, and soon we are chatting about writing and her life as the wife of an Anglican priest. It has not all been easy, she has had a "cross to bear," she says, but it's obvious by the look in her clear blue eyes that she has found a way to interpret her various difficulties in a positive light. Lately she has been helping a close friend of hers die. I sip my wine as she explains that her friend has inoperable cancer of the throat, has maybe three to six months left to live. And then, out of the blue, she says, "But she has faith. She's not at all afraid."

I think how her friend must feel, with death looming inevitably, as her body is slowly weakened and destroyed. Her graceful yielding to her fate is the ultimate acquiescence; she has accepted what will happen to her. She is not interfering or resisting, and so has found solace. The woman and I exchange cards and move on to other people, other conversations.

Next I talk to a small, dark, woman writer, whose husband had died tragically and whose work had been plagiarized. Outwardly she looks so successful: attractive, well-coiffed, charming even. And yet, by her own admission, her inner landscape is a place full of insecurities and mistrust of what life will produce next.

Fresh from my conversation with the priest's wife, I blurt out, "You should have more faith!"

"Oh, but I don't," she sighs. "I'm so afraid."

I can see parts of myself in each of these women. Like the priest's wife, I am aware of faith's power, yet like the widow, I am often too spooked and mesmerized by my own problems to summon it. Perhaps it is not one's circumstances that matter, but rather one's reactions to them. Fear and faith are the fork in the road meeting every traveler.

Guardian Angel

Despite my early training in prayer which consisted mainly of learning to lower my eyes, hold my hands steady before me, and humble myself, I eventually gave up praying to God. That is, I gave up praying directly to God, thinking it wiser to go through the angels. Although angels may seem to be no more than sweetly smiling figures flying happily about, consider for a moment the horrors they have witnessed, the wars, holocausts, famine. Angels serve as the conscience of the ethers; they bear witness.

For years I didn't know enough to pray for the right thing. I recited a litany of wants and needs, a shopping list of desires. I made affirmations. I didn't pray to be healed. I picture the angels like holy stenographers, taking down my requests, their halos radiating with intensity, their eyes so clear that I feel strangely, unnecessarily ashamed in their presence. These days I call upon them often, asking for guidance, for the right thing to happen. I pray for miracles.

Of course, more miracles happen than we recognize. The angels perform fantastic feats regularly, but these feats often go unnoticed. Our lives simply unfold, and in our charmed state, we are oblivious to the dangers that might have befallen us had it not been for the guidance of angels. How many times have we almost suffered a terrible consequence and not even known it? Impossible to count. Angels are always invisibly arriving and departing at just the right time, quietly orchestrating the greater will.

One Halloween Eve, I was driving to San Francisco along busy Bayshore Freeway. Suddenly, the car lost all its power. (I later learned that this was due to a broken timing belt.) While I was aware of the close proximity of the other vehicles speeding past on either side of me and of my own dwindling speed, I knew that I must exit quickly, if only to avoid being hit from behind. This was an instantaneous decision; there wasn't time to think, to wait for a gap in traffic or check the rear-view mirror. "Angels! Help!" I demanded, and I swerved, rolling safely to a stop just inches from calamity.

So I do call upon angels. Angels intrigue me. I often search the sky for a subtle sign that they are there. In her visions, Hildegard of Bingen, the 12th-century mystic, saw angels whose faces reminded her of pure water. "They have wings, not that they are like other winged creatures, but because they fly in their own sphere through the power of God as if they were feathered," Hildegard wrote.

Some believe that we are assigned a guardian angel at birth, whose function is to care for and protect our bodies and souls, to guide us, and to offer our prayers to God.

I wish that I had caught a glimpse of my guardian

angel that night—if only as a slender wing protruding from a shoulder. Instead, I sensed a force-field of benevolence. It was as though everything occurred in an alternate dimension where I simultaneously was and was not, where knives were slow and dull, where time had lost its powers. The air felt magnetic. I know that every atom in the room was changed. The danger of such a reality is that the energy is charged, unpredictable; anything can happen.

I have no doubt that an angel was with me then, sole witness to my terror. There must have been something in the room that shielded me with an armor of unearthly love, using its radiant light to balance darkness.

Spiritual etiquette demands that I now take a quill pen, dip it in the ink of tears, and compose a letter of thanks to my guardian angel. Am I addressing a being clad in robes and halo or something less precise? It doesn't matter. What I experienced that night was so far beyond the mundane, the material, that I can be sure of nothing less than that this entity is beyond my imagination.

Still, I picture my guardian angel sitting cross-legged by a river, wings draped behind him. There is no need to explain who I am or why I've come. He knows. Spirits have an intimacy that bodies will never know.

Thanking one of God's messengers requires a shift in consciousness. There is a cynical part of me that is aware that I wouldn't be giving thanks if something terrible hadn't happened, and so I resent it. Still, I *am* grateful. And the words "thank you" alone seem hollow.

Guardian Angel

Dear Guardian Angel,

It is strange not to know by name the one who rescued me from death's whirlpool, that steady, benevolent figure who offered me a point of calm in the midst of terror and chaos, whose wings were drawn around me, forming a shield. By your radiance alone, I was spared. It was your curious light that captured my attention, distracting me, drawing me toward it.

That night, you stopped time by mesmerizing the hands of clocks until the minutes and hours meant nothing.

You held one finger against the knife's glinting tip, making it powerless.

You heard the scream that never left my throat.

You saw my trembling self.

You witnessed what we all, together, could not see.

You swayed in the balmy breeze which blew the curtains.

You whispered to each man, reminding him of his conscience.

You forgave each man his fear and greed and ignorance when he didn't listen.

You stayed near.

You said a prayer that echoes yet.

You felt their strength.

You accepted as though it were a gift their violent desire.

You sacrificed innocence, which they destroyed.

You moved among us with watery gentleness.

You shone like a star that perpetually rises and never leaves the sky.

You absorbed the pain.

Later, you held evil in your gentle arms, transforming it.

You cried for them.

You have always been with me, are with me still, quietly guiding, protecting, looking out for my welfare. For all these reasons, and more, I give my thanks.

Synchronicity

Tonight is the twenty-fourth anniversary of the rape. That night, all those years ago, she was sitting at a typewriter, composing poems. The incident that would radically change her life hadn't happened yet. These pieces of time dance inside my mind, disjointed, like clumsy puppets.

I see her writing in darkness, alone, hypnotized by words, but with no real knowledge of danger. The warning flows through her unrecognized. I see her go upstairs, turning toward the window with a gesture of nonchalance. She is still innocent. She can trust the night. Then she undresses, gets into bed. Maybe she has a twinge of apprehension as she closes her eyes. I want to tell her that, though she will pass through a trial, she will be safe. Yet she cannot hear me. As she drifts to sleep, dissolving in a dream, as the room becomes silent but for her breaths, I must wait and watch. The moon through the gauzy orange curtains casts a soft light upon her sleeping figure. She bathes in the lunar glow, absorbing moonbeams into her sleeping body so young and full.

The echo of her inverse scream, the scream that never was, reaches me now. But it is too late. The men are already there, the knife is raised. It seems possible that the black hole of death might suck her in, and all that has occurred between then and now trail behind her in a vapor of what-ifs.

Yet somehow I have arrived safely on the other side of that calamity. The two are gone, though for twenty-four years I have lugged their ghostly weight as an invisible burden.

You can leave a place, but a place never leaves you.

I decide to mark the anniversary of the night I almost died, when my soul was dislocated from the rest of me. I need a ritual, but short of lighting a candle and gazing at its small flame, I have none. Besides, I'm restless. So instead I approach the meandering roads of London as though they are the circuits of a labyrinth.

As I walk, I ask for a sign. I haven't gone far, a hundred paces or so, when I come across a large picture in a gold frame discarded on the sidewalk. The palm trees first snare my attention, then the sandy beach, the aqua sky. It is a picture of Hawaii—strangely exotic and yet at the same time homely—like one might find in a travel agent's office.

Usually just the mention of the word "Hawaii" causes me to experience an inward cringe, a chill of fear, but now, perhaps owing to my questing mood, my recent airing of memories, and my compulsion to put those memories into words, I feel unmoved.

As I turn my head sideways to further examine the picture, I notice two men lumbering down the road toward me. Although I'd like to share my discovery, they have about them a hostile air. Oddly, they seem not to notice me or the incongruous tropical scene propped against its backdrop of London.

Once they pass, I feel a bittersweet smile come to my lips. The picture is a gift of sorts, the angels' way of saying, "See? It's just an old discarded image now. It can't harm you anymore."

Synchronicities such as this—"inexplicable meaningful coincidences"—are, for me, moments of grace. Sprinkled like breadcrumbs along the path of my life, they have served to fill me with awe and amusement, leading me, step by step, back to a place of faith and trust in the universal unfolding.

That is not to say that I do not often slip and fall and curse the chaos. Because I do. As I've said, it is always a struggle between fear and faith, and quite often fear wins. Yet it is helpful sometimes to remember that these magical links do exist and, while often well-hidden, are always accessible. It seems that they are generously provided for us (often when we least expect them) by a playful, benevolent force.

Jung coined the term synchronicity to explain the "psychic parallelisms which cannot be related to each other causally" (that is, by the law of cause and effect). Think of a child's connect-the-dots drawing. One dot leads logically to the other, but the white space between the dots is where the mystery resides. That white space is the plane on which synchronicities—in the form of dreams, visions, or actual events—occur.

I had a friend who was always experiencing synchronicities. My phone would ring, and it would be her, exclaiming, "You won't believe what just happened!" Many times our individual synchronicities overlapped, leaving us stunned and full of wonder. Overwhelmed by their frequency and sensing a trend, she began recording every detail, describing events along with her revelations, in page after page of a handwritten journal. This kept her so busy that while the synchronicities continued, she was eventually forced to abandon her recording of them.

These often bewildering experiences are said to result from an inner psychic image that is inexplicably mirrored by an outer event. It is interesting to note that according to Jung's colleague, the analyst Aniela Jaffé, "synchronistic phenomena are most likely to occur in the vicinity of archetypal happenings like death, deadly danger, catastrophes, crises, upheavals, etc." I have found that the opposite is also true: I become a magnet for such happenings when I am at my most open and joyful.

Jung addressed the mystery of these coincidences when he wrote the following.

Meaningful coincidences are thinkable as pure chance....But the more they multiply and the greater and more exact the correspondence is, the more their probability sinks and their unthinkability increases, until they can no longer be regarded as pure chance but, for lack of a causal explanation, have to be thought of as meaningful arrangements....Their 'inexplicability' *is not due to the fact that the cause is unknown, but to the fact that a cause is not even thinkable in intellectual terms.*

I'll leave the last word to Julian of Norwich, the 14th-century saint and mystic. During a serious illness, Julian received a number of visions. In order to meditate on these "shewings," she sequestered herself in a cell for twenty years. She then wrote about her visions in *Revelations of Divine Love*. To her, synchronicities were purely the work of God.

And I saw that nothing happens by chance, but by the far-sighted wisdom of God. If it seems like chance to us, it is because we are blind and blinkered.

The things planned before the world began come upon us suddenly, so that in our blindness we say that they are chance. But God knows better. Constantly and lovingly he brings all that happens to its best end.

For Mary Hearthern

Writing this book has been like mending from the inside out. I have felt a sense of release, an unburdening, a relief to finally tell the truth. It has been like one great sigh in words.

My compulsion to put these words to paper occurred as naturally as a change of seasons. There was no choice, just as in spring, a tree's leaves are born from dormant wood or a flower effortlessly opens its fan of colorful petals. Suddenly it didn't matter what people thought or whether they saw me differently than before. Perhaps I would be pitied. I didn't care. As I scribbled notes, I became aware that there might be an even worse consequence for *not* telling. I needed to uncover, reclaim, move forward. Like Scheherazade, my motivation was one of self-preservation.

Scheherazade told her stories to entertain her new husband, with the aim of surviving yet another night. Hadn't he done away with all his previous wives? The sands sifting through the hourglass meant everything to her. Each story had to be totally captivating and unique and yet each shared a common purpose—to save her from strangulation by the sultan. Imagine trying to simultaneously entrance and enlighten such a man! Yet even more was at stake: Each time she succeeded in seducing him with words, she not only saved her own life, but she also saved the lives of those women who would have otherwise inevitably followed her as the sultan's wife. The pressure, therefore, was great.

I also needed to accept and honor what had happened on another level. For it was not just about rape; it was also about divine intervention, a seeing between worlds, an initiation.

Buddhist teacher Pema Chödrön points out that our messy lives are fertile territory for new growth. It is up to us to use them that way. This is what I have tried to do.

I don't know that I'll ever forgive, though maybe, by writing this, I have already begun—if only by forgiving myself. I will never know who I might be today if that incident hadn't happened. That robbing of my potential self was the greatest rape of all. I may have triumphed by my survival of it, but even that act has forever changed me.

Before the rape, Hawaii was simply a distant, sunny place to go on vacation. I once painted a watercolor of two hula dancers waving at a man on a sailboat. It is unclear whether he is in distress, shipwrecked, arriving or departing. This fragment of paradise has survived, reminding me of that time, the time *before*.

Another artifact from back then was displayed for

many years in my old bedroom at my parent's house. It was a photograph of me as a teenager in Maui, posing in front of the ocean in my bikini. I'm smiling. What's interesting is that my feet are cut from the frame, giving me an unrooted appearance. It was the only picture of me, and one of but a few well-chosen decorations in their sparsely furnished home. Every time I saw it, I'd wonder, How could that experience [of the rape] *not* have shattered me? How could that smiling young girl ever survive it?

In reality, my twenty-year-old self couldn't do much more than bury her fear and anger, and try to get on with her life. I forgive her for returning to her job at the department store, where, "floating" from department to department, she again sold chocolate turtles and tennis rackets, measured yards of fabric, and knelt before children, fitting their tiny feet with shoes—all as if nothing had happened. I forgive her for her romantic escapades, going from man to man as though she were dancing the Virginia Reel. If she behaved promiscuously, it is hard to say whether it was in keeping with the pleasure-seeking times or a fallout from the rape, for paradoxically, such behavior can be an unconscious way of desensitizing oneself to sex, taking away its meaning and its power. I forgive her for her sadness, her anxiety attacks, and her inability to ever again see the world as a safe place.

I am ashamed, though, that I was not sufficiently aware and brave enough to return to Hawaii and prosecute them. I know that some women, willing to continue facing their trauma, take their fight to the courts, experiencing victory when the perpetrator is given a prison sentence—

and paranoia if he is released. I cannot imagine the dread one must feel then. I wanted to end my karma with my assailants. And I knew that prison isn't going to stop rape; only human consciousness can. Seeing them behind bars wouldn't have made me feel any better, though it would have prevented those two particular men from raping again—for a time.

Besides, I knew nothing about the legal system, save what I'd garnered from watching Perry Mason on TV, and there was no "support network" to speak of. There was only me, and revenge was not a strong enough trait in my young heart. It is unfortunate that I even feel the need to supply an excuse, as though the responsibility for their behavior was, and is, my own.

Yet I do hope that, like Scheherazade's, my words will serve some purpose. While multitudes of women have been raped, few ever speak of it. The vocabulary of rape, I discovered, is full of blind spots. Much is said about the rapist, his background, and what causes a man to rape (from a woman's provocative dress to the influences of the media). This was made clear to me when I was browsing in the British Library and found a book published in 1823. The flyleaf read: "From The Life, Character and Conduct of William Biggs, who was executed at the last Gloucester Assizes, for having committed a rape, robbery, and murder, on the body of Mary Hearthern."

On the body of...

It implies that she was no more than that, a mere vessel to receive the inevitable evil. A sacrifice. It is all about him, this William Biggs. What about her? Mary

Hearthern's story is the one I want to hear. Who was she? What did she feel in those moments before she died? Does her spirit rest, or does it still flutter, distressed?

Stray Arrows

I may not know why the rape occurred, whether it was accidental or whether it served some higher purpose. Yet, by seeing it as more than a criminal assault, I am, at least, offered a balm for my startled self. For it was the divine that indelibly touched me, not the bruise left by Hyena and Dark One. Their physical violence was like a roving shadow compared to the great transforming jolt received by my psyche. Over time, I have come to understand that if something that terrible could happen, then so could something equally as miraculous.

I was lucky: I lived. I have the opportunity to tell my story, the luxury to forgive. Forgiving Hyena and Dark One is one thing; I still struggle with that process. Forgiving Simon, on the other hand, is even harder than forgiving myself.

Although it is easy to trace the incident back to Simon as source, I know in my heart that he never intended anything bad to happen to me, and that he was probably as destroyed by his own guilt as he was by that evening's violence. Still, he didn't protect me (though his passivity may have played a part in our survival). So I suppose I am angry. By his absence in my life, he has remained an elusive character and so my feelings toward him are often misplaced, like stray arrows.

When I think of Simon now, I see him in the field, pausing by the twisted grey oak of my childhood. Oddly, the photograph I had taken of him that day never turned out. Yet it is as if the image were burned into my soul. I can see his great black hat, his pensive stare. Perhaps, like Oscar Wilde, he also held his hand over his heart. Recently I learned that Oscar Wilde had kept company with a prostitute, who was later murdered. He wrote a poem, inspired by her, called "The Harlot's House": *"...the dead are dancing with the dead / the dust is whirling with the dust..."*

Will I ever see him again? Maybe. But I think not.

Rainbow

The day beckons. I stop writing and walk down a long, tree-lined lane in Regent's Park. I notice a small girl balanced in the crotch of one of the trees. Like an owl, her steely eyes gaze out with brave certainty. Merging with the world in such a way, half-visible, half-hidden, she seems to draw power not only from what is known, but rather from all that is unknown and, therefore, possible.

The one time I climbed a tree, I happened to sample a poisonous, chartreuse-colored berry while in its boughs. As I bit into the hard, bitter, astringent fruit, I felt a curious rush of fear, just as Persephone might have done, when she tasted the first pomegranate seed of the underworld. Yet this girl in Regent's Park is brave; she is intent to climb still higher. She shifts position to survey the dappled green overhead. And then she shimmies up, disappearing into a web of leaves and brittle branches.

Although the humid weather is stifling, there is also something soothing about it, luxurious almost.

Everyone has discarded their heavy winter coats and scarves, revealing their pale shoulders. They all move in slow motion. I also deliberately slow my pace, stopping to appreciate the simplicity of the clouds hanging in the sky like metallic-grey prayer flags. It has been raining on and off all day, as it begins to now.

Then a rainbow appears. It hovers over a playing field, near the not-so-distant horizon. I begin walking toward it. The rainbow dips behind a tree, where a small group of people huddle. How strange that they cannot see it, but rather only curse the rain as they cling to the one umbrella between them.

With my rainbow clearly in sight, I don't care that my shoes are wet or that my cotton trousers are drooping like water-laden tulips. I am only aware of my bliss. The weather is warm and balmy, the trees lush; there is a lazy, gentle feeling in the scented air. Then I realize—this weather reminds me of Hawaii.

Not the Hawaii that I knew in April of 1976, but the Hawaii before that, when nothing terrible had happened to me and, it seemed, never would. The Hawaii of my girlhood. Memories of its natural beauty and kitschy charm come flooding back to me along with the groggy, seductive scent of pineapples and men in luau shirts.

For the first time in years, I am able to appreciate Hawaii for what it was and what I suppose still is—a paradise. Never mind that its archipelago of misty islands once towered above the ocean as moody volcanic mountains and that its waterfalls, by virtue of their mystery, were even more enchanted. Never mind that its original inhabitants were not intruded upon by tourists. Yes, there is something about that place which I still love and which will always be a part of me.

Radiant colors arc above. Red, orange, yellow... And then I see it, not too far from where I stand: the rainbow's end.

Or is it its beginning?

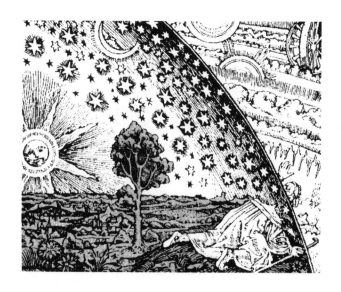

Prayer

Courage is fear, which has said its prayers. I recall this old Huguenot epitaph as I find some matches and light a votive candle. Soon the room is scented with honeysuckle, sweet heather, rose, and peppermint. I summon the angels—or at least, try to. *Are you there?* I ask, hopeful and expectant.

I wait for a clue, a rustle or a wavering motion at the periphery of my vision.

There is no answer, only the chiming birdsong outside, that single fading melody, which sounds and then dissolves in the silver evening sky.

Drawing the drapes, I sit on a chair and place my opened hands on my lap. I lower my eyes. That sparkling blue cross, relic of childhood, calls to me now, just as it called to me then. Yet tonight I will forgo the formalities of prayer that Reverend McConnell tried so patiently to teach me.

Instead, I become still and journey to the divine

within myself. While I'm meditating, I imagine a taproot anchoring me to the center of the earth, and a golden web rising from my head to the heavens. Connected to the universe in this manner, I am everything and nothing in the dreamy landscape of my inner darkness.

Within the quiet of my heart, a seed of compassion breaks open. A lavish, abundant bloom fills me with its gentle petals. And so, I say a prayer for all of us—for those who have raped or been raped, for those who have been betrayed, humiliated, controlled, attacked, and for those who have played the part of villain in that drama. I say a prayer for the healing of every injustice that has ever occurred since the beginning of time and for every injustice that will occur at some future date. And, knowing that pain and suffering have no real gauge by which to measure them, I say a prayer for the little girl I saw crying near the Royal Observatory in Greenwich, so caught was she in some fragile drama that her anguished expression has stuck with me. Her tears are no less relevant than the ones I would also cry, if I could. All tears come from the same source.

I gaze for a while at the candle, as its blue core holds still in the dancing flame. And then I gently blow it out.

So be it.

This is my story, my thousand-and-one nights. Its twists and turns are not so important; what matters is that I have told it, and you have listened.

Part IV

And the end of all our exploring
Will be to arrive where we started
And know the place for the first time.

T.S. ELIOT

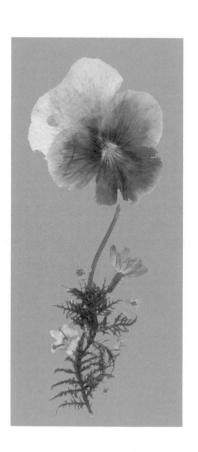

Pilgrimage

Much has happened since I wrote those last words. Finally, my story was on the page. Seeing it as a truth—however painful—*outside* myself, and gaining perspective as I shared it with others, I gradually began to feel more distance. This type of writing (known as scriptotherapy, *writing as healing*) stirred up my psyche, to be sure, but it was also liberating and desensitized me to some of the rape's harmful memories.

It can be profoundly transforming to put into words the previously hidden aspects of one's psyche. As writer May Sarton discovered, "To close the door on pain is to miss the chance for growth." Truth is power.

It was for me. The book that you are now holding in your hands is my testimony of that.

Scriptotherapy works by linking memories of an event with corresponding emotions. These emotions relate to one's feelings both then *and* now. For example, in my writing about Hawaii, I described my feelings at the time of the incident as well as my feelings about that incident now. This created a useful bridge between past and present. Crossing it, I was able to return to the maiden in me and honor her feelings. On the bridge's other side I was able to view the maiden from the woman's perspective, which, in turn, made it possible for me to recognize the present moment, to catch up to real time. By anchoring the book in childhood, I accessed a "pure" time, a time "before," which gave me a counterbalance for the sadness and shame I now felt. These different aspects of myself—the girl, the maiden, and the woman—were important in my personal integration. I needed all three working together on the page in order to grow and heal.[1]

Since it was the labyrinth walk at Grace Cathedral that millennium's eve that had given me the inspiration and courage to write *Risk to Blossom* in the first place, and since writing had brought to light a dark and cloistered part of myself, I came to believe that writing and walking together could benefit others as well. Researching the history of labyrinths, learning from facilitators, and relying on my own soul knowledge, I created WordWalk.

In the WordWalk workshops, walking and writing are solitary yet shared acts which bring us to a place deep within ourselves. Walking in silent meditation, we each come into synch with the fragile, imperfect (yet paradoxically perfect), wondrous journey of our life. Linked writing rituals (such as spirit names, stream-of-consciousness, letter writing, and affirmations) explore the stories of our uncensored hearts, whether they tell of trauma or joy. During this process, personal truth and authenticity spring up like wildflowers in a field. It's that simple and that complex.

Tapping into these two activities can provide some illuminating insights. This is especially so if one is at a crossroads. "Where am I on the path of my life?" one might ask. "Where have I been, and where am I going?"

Traveling about with a Chartres-style, purple-painted canvas labyrinth along with a bag of colored pens and paper, I visited different spiritual groups and communities in England and the States, giving WordWalk workshops and "open walks" (in which anyone was welcome to participate). It was a magic carpet ride of possibilities.

While my intention was to be of service, ironically I was also doing what was hardest for me: staying in one strange place after another, adapting to a series of lumpy duvets, idiosyncratic tea-makers, and broken boilers. Some restless nights I lay awake, listening for creaking floorboards. No sooner had I "settled" than I was off again, maneuvering my suitcase, cumbersome labyrinth, and laptop computer in and out of lifts and up and down spiral staircases. For someone who had previously avoided traveling, now I was unstoppable. Like my Romanian gypsy ancestors, I tried to adhere to the principles of most wandering peoples—"lightness, courtesy, alertness, and solidarity"— but somehow the concept of traveling light always seemed to evade me.

During my very first workshop, a parade marched by outside the rented hall, shattering the meditative silence. At the Palm Sunday event (on the rape's 25th anniversary) in the St. James's Church courtyard in Piccadilly with its blooming magnolia, the customary donkey was not allowed to attend because of the outbreak of foot-and-mouth disease. Days earlier, I had felt as though I were smuggling in contraband goods and not a spiritual healing tool as I passed through customs with my labyrinth, which was no more than ground covering to them and therefore, in light of the current epidemic, a potential health risk and confiscatable.

I had become a pilgrim, if sometimes a reluctant one. Still, I persevered.

I boomeranged many times across the Atlantic. There was one journey I dreaded, though I wasn't sure why. Even as I packed, I suffered crying jags. Something felt not quite right.

My trip had already been delayed once because of mundane reasons involving my host's new kitchen floor (the glue needed to dry before anyone walked on the tiles). Then I missed the next flight out, only to find, after waiting at the airport, that the other two flights were full. I decided to rest over the weekend. With any luck, I'd still be in London by Tuesday, in enough time for a weekend Open Walk that I was presenting.

Flying standby can be a trying experience. Again, I waited at the departure gate, clutching my carry-on, not knowing what would happen, whether I would go or be sent back home again. My name was the last one called.

After the long flight (during which I was seated in the center of Economy between a child and his Game Boy and an irritable Irishwoman), I arrived jet-lagged in London, only to discover that my baggage—including the labyrinth— had been lost.[2] It seemed a great disaster.

That same day I was faced with the events of September 11th. As the story unfolded and the world froze with shock and then grief, I understood that I was on no ordinary journey.

This time, however, I was not alone in my fears. There was evil in the hearts of some and uncertainty was most definitely in the air. As the leaders of countries seemed unable to find humane solutions to ancient problems, it became clear to me that we are all—even in our ordinary, often anonymous lives—the caretakers of this planet. Heeding our hearts as we move forward together into the unknown, our test will be to choose the path of faith, not fear. Now, we are all pilgrims.

Introducing the labyrinth to others became a passion. I loved hearing the revelations after a walk, aware of the miraculous inner changes that had occurred. Those who seemed skeptical at first were often the ones who ended up crying. Revelations flowed. One participant learned how a feeling of gratitude leads the way to humility. Others said they felt blessed or peaceful. The labyrinth's power was undeniable.

Yet how the labyrinth actually works remains a mystery. Some say that the brain's left and right hemispheres are balanced during a labyrinth walk. Inherent in the act of pacing itself is the calming tonic of thoughtfulness and introspection, which make it a suitable antidote for the "millennial fatigue" brought on by a fast-forwarded lifestyle in danger of losing its connection to the past. Whatever the reason, there is something about the labyrinth that strongly resonates with the human spirit.

Even so, the act of going inward may be fraught with some anxiety, especially for those of us who have experienced trauma in our lives. We are afraid of what Minotaur awaits us; it seems easier to turn away. One thing I have discovered from working with the labyrinth as a spiritual tool is that we all have hidden vulnerabilities that hold us back from the natural blossoming that is our birthright. By not acknowledging our weaknesses, by hiding too well those wounds from others (and, more crucially, from ourselves), we cannot fully *own* our corresponding strength. This can be addressed, a step at a time, by following the labyrinth's soul-mirroring path.

Thomas Merton wrote, "The geographical pilgrimage is the symbolic acting out of an inner journey." Labyrinth walks are little pilgrimages in disguise. In the labyrinth's healing vessel, we are led to the sacredness within ourselves, and thus, to an awareness of the sacredness of the greater world. Like a pilgrimage, a labyrinth walk involves going away from or toward a place or state of being. There is often an element of synchronicity found in a labyrinth walk, a feeling that one is on an uncommonly meaningful, if beguiling journey. It is as though reality has shifted ever so slightly, giving one the sensation of being happily lost in unfamiliar territory.

---

[1]"Give sorrow words: The grief that does not speak whispers the over-wrought heart, and bids it break." (Shakespeare)

[2]Thankfully, later everything was returned to me.

Mapping the Invisible

How does one heal? Although there is no map to follow and ultimately each must make her or his own way (while calling on others for support), I have found that there are three basic energetic tools which can help navigate the healing journey: acceptance, willingness, and compassion.

ACCEPTANCE. While truth is often as hard to bear as the incident itself, living under false pretenses serves no one. It only perpetuates another lie, which yearns to be unraveled. By keeping my secret, I made the mistake of trying to live like other people and did not live like me. For the teller of any lie there is always a psychic toll.

I have learned that one must accept what has happened. This means looking at the scars and shadows, which are precisely what you do not want to see. By revisiting a past traumatic event with the purpose of honoring it, a separation occurs between you and it. You begin to trust that it is not happening *now*. This gives you perspective and, eventually, some neutrality. It roots you safely in the present moment. This is true only if you dare to look; otherwise you will always be denying, avoiding, running from it, and it will continue to have its phantom's power over you.

Of course, there are positive aspects as well. That you survived, for instance. And, in doing so, have gained a depth of soul and character. You cannot change what has happened (nor is it necessary to condone it), yet you can choose to see *your* truth in a new way. By gradually letting go of the victim consciousness within yourself, you become a heroine. Your sights are set on strength, not weakness. Moving through pain, you learn to use it, rather than letting the pain use you. An excellent way of doing this is by channeling pain into art.

WILLINGNESS. This is about openness and vulnerability—the risk to blossom. Uncomfortable as this risk may feel, it does clear a space for healing. The discomfort involved in healing is ultimately of greater benefit—and thus perhaps more bearable—than the discomfort of staying stuck.

Opening to the present moment helps to release and/or integrate some of your negative feelings such as anger, resentment, and fear. Of course, there is a time for turning inward and processing pain (I picture a hedgehog, curled in on itself). Healing can also occur with no effort on your part. However, by setting your intention (for example, affirming, "I am open to the spirit of healing"), you naturally attract to you the people and circumstances and lessons that you need, and, perhaps even more important, you are more apt to recognize them when they appear.

Additionally, by surrendering to a Higher Power (if you believe in one) or "casting the burden on the Christ within," as Florence Scovel Shinn advises in *The Game of Life*, you are freed on an even deeper level. The prayer "Thy will be done" is very liberating. "Thy" here refers to God or Allah, the *tao* (the way), the inconceivable, regenerative, universal force, which has fueled our human drama since the beginning of time. Yet even with the blessing of divine assistance, you must still participate in your own healing.

Recovering from a crisis such as rape does not happen all at once. It takes time.

COMPASSION. Search your heart for what it most resists—for instance, someone who has deeply hurt you—and you will discover where your compassion is most needed. If you can try to imagine what it might be like to walk the sometimes smooth, sometimes rocky path of another's reality, you will be that much closer to finding compassion, as well as the qualities of forgiveness and love, within yourself.

Compassion (from the Latin *com* or "with" and *pati*, "to suffer") is about feeling the suffering of others, suffering *with* them. Of course, the deeper your own pain, the easier it is to recognize it in someone else. By honoring any pain in a non-judgmental way, you draw healing to it. All suffering beings deserve such consideration.

The art of compassion is found in the selfless opening to the universal pain for the sake of another. It is sympathy and caring sent where it is needed. If you have difficulty offering compassion to someone who has betrayed, humiliated, controlled, attacked, or hurt you in some way, start with someone you genuinely like. Can you identify with a misfortune in her or his life? From there, expand that feeling to include family and neighbors, friends and strangers.[3] Consider too the billions of inhabitants of this fragile world whose conditions seem hopeless and unfair, especially those who are deemed useless and unworthy. Now turn back to the one you cannot forgive. Compassion is the arrow of the heart that pierces the most difficult target. It is the ability to see within the "enemy" a vulnerable piece of yourself, to love (or try to, anyway) that which is hardest, if not impossible, to fathom. Compassion asks you to be greater and stronger than you are until you become just that.

For it is both a sorry consolation and a fact of life that in your pain you are not alone. Tears flood the planet. You can chose to ignore them, or you can realize that any tear shed by another belongs to you as well. True compassion is unconditional. By becoming a channel of healing, you are also healed.

"My grievances hide the light of the world in me," states *A Course in Miracles*. Compassion is a step toward reversing that darkness and reclaiming light. It is a healing, alchemical dance. Acting from a place of compassion, you create a new flow of energy within and without yourself. Then anger, resentment, and fear can become peace, forgiveness, and faith. This leads to an appreciation of the sweetness of life, a treasuring of all its ordinary and extraordinary moments. And a strong sense of gratitude. You cannot feel like a victim, *and* give thanks; gratitude is empowering.

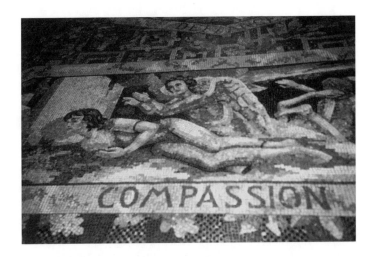

While I have applied my approach of acceptance, willingness, and compassion to the rape experience in particular, it is also useful when healing from other types of traumas and diseases of the spirit.

Mapping your own healing path can be both difficult and wondrous. Sometimes it may seem lonely; other times not so, as you join with other travelers. It is helpful to let go of how you think the path should unfold and to simply make a commitment to follow it. As Lao Tzu said, "The longest journey begins with a single step."

As part of this process, you may want to create your own healing rituals. Finding a sacred space where you will be undisturbed, you can simply do what feels appropriate for you. For example, you might light a candle, sing a healing song, dance under the full moon, or bless yourself with sacred water.

Another spiritual tool that must be mentioned is intuition, the language of the unconscious or the inner guidance that manifests as dreams, hunches, and visions. Oddly practical, it hints and warns, aiding survival. It is important to learn this language, to heed its message. You can call upon your higher knowing right now by using the following visualization.

Close your eyes and imagine an old medicine woman seated before you. She wears a ceremonial dress the color of dreams, and a cap of shells and feathers. The sound of her small round drum is like the soothing rhythm of heartbeats. There is something strong and wise and familiar about her. You feel at ease in her presence and sense that she is there to help you. Now she reaches inside her supple leather pouch, where she finds amongst its treasures a special healing object that is meant for you. She offers it to you with a blessing. What is it? What do you need for your journey?

The journey of healing is often very long. There is no moment when all is magically forgiven and forgotten, the fear erased, and the unclean past made pristine. Yet, in the act of journeying, you continually remake and reinvent yourself, becoming far more than your pain ever was.

---

[3]I remember my mother befriending a tearful young woman in the Greyhound bus depot in Sacramento, California. With forlorn-looking suitcase and rumpled coat, it seemed as though the woman were running from something or someone, and my mother was there, asking if she needed help, gently probing. Ironically, it was from my mother that I first learned about the art of compassion.

$\mathcal{P}$ersephone's $\mathcal{R}$eturn

There is a 4th-century B.C. painting found in a royal tomb which shows Persephone's abduction by the god of the underworld. Much of the scene is obscured, and just one of Persephone's round, frightened eyes is still visible in the coarse and faded image that has survived. It is a haunting reminder of the reality of rape. She seems to be calling out to us across the centuries.

Her expression serves as a mirror to all rape survivors. For, in her plight, that frozen moment of consequence when she was seized by Hades (otherwise she would have just gone on frolicking in the field) we see ourselves. Something terrible is happening: She is broken and ruined; she does not pretend to be whole, nor can onlookers who are uncomfortable with violence be shielded from her truth. Yet even by her suffering, she does not endorse the "privilege" of forever feeling sorry for ourselves. Persephone's mythic power, her gift to us, is her ability to descend to the very depths of adversity and then to rise up from it, no longer maiden, now goddess. Hers is not an easy path, but it is one of power. By her survival, Persephone shows us how we, too, can reclaim the goddesses within ourselves.

For what is a goddess, really, but one who is in touch with all the aspects of herself? The pain and fury as well as the wisdom and courage. She isn't perfect; in fact, she is often profoundly flawed with a burden (or two) to bear. When a wounded woman chooses to be, not a victim, but a goddess in spirit, the world changes. Authentic feminine energies are restored, given voice, and unleashed. Her impact cannot be ignored. It is impossible to shrink back and accept a world that has been defined for centuries by men, when that world is in the process of being destroyed. Something else is needed to bring it into balance. Hers is a different way. For her to discover it, she must first find and accept and honor herself. She needs to see clearly through that eye of horror and discern good from bad, light from dark, so that she can move forward. Only then will there be balance in her own heart and in that of the world.

Sometimes it seems that there is no vessel deep enough to hold our tears, no magic remedy to cure our psychic wounds. Certainly nothing will ever take away the shock, the horror, the injustice. And yet, these tragedies can become our greatest teachers.

To those who have had similar experiences as mine, my message is as follows: Feel the pain. Own it. Learn from it. Forgive, if you can. And know that you are not alone. The repercussions of rape can be transformed into something good and powerful in your life. With grace, even the most potent curse can become a blessing.

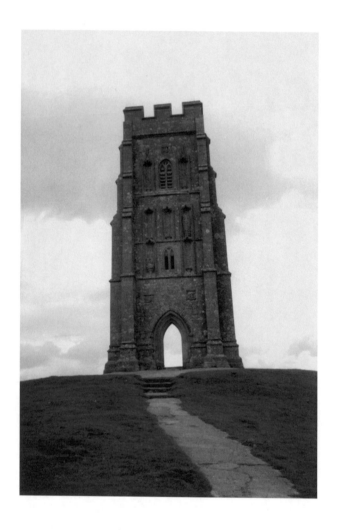

Chalice Well Gardens

Eight months after the World Trade Center came falling down like the burning tower in the tarot cards, I have made yet another journey. This time, after traveling by car and plane and cab and tube and train and bus and, of course, by foot, I finally reach Glastonbury, a town in Mendip, Somerset, in southwest England. The occasion is The Labyrinth Society's first international symposium. England, Scotland, Wales, France, the United States, the Netherlands, Sweden, Switzerland, Austria, Germany, Portugal, and Israel are among the countries represented. I am here to learn more about labyrinths and to meet others involved in this work. Some heavy-duty bonding is occurring as an abundance of arcane information, stories, and visions are shared. I should have known that this might happen, given the labyrinth's way of stirring up synchronicities and its uncanny ability to "meet you where you are and give you what you need." Then too, Glastonbury is linked to legends both Christian and

Arthurian. It is where Joseph of Arimathea is believed to have brought the chalice from the Last Supper. King Arthur (of the Round Table and the Holy Grail) and his Queen Guinevere are said to be buried on the grounds of the mystical, if desolate Abbey.

I am staying at Pilgrims B&B, at the home of a woman named Koko. With soft brown eyes and a radiant smile, she tells me she is a healer. She does soul retrieval. *Hmmm...soul retrieval? Sounds intense,* I think, gripping my suitcase. I had been warned that everyone in this town is into something "New Agey," and there are more shops selling crystals than basics like milk and bread. Now I have firsthand experience. I only hope that she can make a decent breakfast with not-too-runny eggs and that there are enough blankets for the bed.

I follow her up the stairs. When she opens the door to the room I am to stay in (which belongs to her son, who is off traveling in India), I am immediately taken aback by the many posters on the walls—all surfers. High waves, sandy beaches, half-naked young men. I am instantly reminded of Hawaii. Perhaps because our timing was off earlier and I had been kept waiting outside for an hour-and-a-half making small talk with a Reiki master, I'm tired, in need of a cup of tea and a shower, and my resistance to such things is low.

"Is something wrong?" asks Koko.

"Yes, I mean no, it's just that—." I look with searching eyes at all the posters, at her, and back at the posters. "Is there, uh, another room?" But she's full up because of the labyrinth symposium; this room is the only one left.

"No worries," she says simply. "My son won't care. I'll just take them down." And, to my amazement, she begins methodically removing all the posters from the walls. Because there are so many of them, I help her by yanking down a few too. *Be gone, Hyena. Be gone, Dark One*, I think with a sigh. Now the walls are bare. It feels good.

Spring. Time of rebirth and renewal. When Persephone ascends from the darkness of the underworld. The fields and hills of Glastonbury are a brilliant, vibrant green. Wildflowers sway under wind and sudden showers. This is when the Celtic season of Beltane begins. When the May tree works its wonders. It is a sacred time.

Chalice Well Gardens, known as a natural shrine, has been a place of pilgrimage for thousands of years. A healing spring flows from this site, which stands in the shadow of the ancient Tor. A canvas labyrinth has been arranged on the lawn, and a woman is gently gathering us together, offering her hand and dancing up the slopes in a chain of silent people.

Soon I am among them, flowing past a blur of greenery and by-now-familiar faces. When it comes time to form a circle around the labyrinth, a few of us are already in tears. Watching the others as they begin to walk, I become aware of their fragility and transparency. With each person's footfall, I sense my own joy and pain. It becomes clear to me that we are all connected in ways we will probably never fully understand. It is a miracle that we are here, in this Eden of possibilities, meeting on this sacred path. This moment is a gift.

Overhead, birds circle around and around, as

though to mirror us. While I wait my turn, I try to process my myriad feelings. All I know is that if I feel any more, I will erupt in tears that may never stop—like the water that has ceaselessly flowed from the Chalice Well for centuries.

Taking refuge under a willow tree, I consider my past, its weak spots and its strengths. My life has been a labyrinth of mysterious turnings and tests and magic. Along the way, I have met my share of angels and Minotaurs— and, thinking of my room back at the B&B, even a few modern-day shamans. Yet however circuitous my life may appear, I have the feeling that I have at last arrived somewhere. It is as though all my journeying has led me to this one place, this healing spot. Here, all my different selves meet: the girl who danced the May Pole Dance, the child who ran from her father in search of some evasive truth, the one who sat so solemnly in a druidic circle of stones—and the woman with her nightmarish past, her Scheherazade's tales.

I gaze up at the gentle English sky. Maybe my soul has been retrieved, after all.

ⓦhat Ⓘ Ⓑelieve

✢ *I believe in a Higher Power in which I, Nature, the stars, and all creation are a part.*

✢ *I believe that the soul does not die.*

✢ *I believe that we are ultimately held accountable, whether in this life or the next, for our thoughts, actions, and deeds.*

✢ *I believe that while all is in a constant state of change, a balance of primal opposites is maintained.*

✢ *I believe that there will always be a mystery beyond our comprehension.*

✢ *I believe that love does, indeed, make the world go 'round.*

Works Cited

PART I

Epigraph. Mirabai, in *Women in Praise of the Sacred*, ed. by Jane Hirshfield (New York: HarperCollins, 1994), p. 132.

PART II

Epigraph. H.D. (Hilda Doolittle), *Helen in Egypt* (New York: New Directions, 1974), p. 116. Randy Thornhill and Craig T. Palmer, *A Natural History of Rape: Biological Bases of Sexual Coercion* (Cambridge, MA: The MIT Press, 2001), pp. ? Eckhart Tolle, *The Power of Now: A Guide to Spiritual Enlightenment*, pp. 27-38. "Little Brown Gal" lyrics and music copyright © 1935 by Don McDiarmid and Lee Wood. Traumatic Stress Clinic, *Psychological Reactions to Trauma* (London: Traumatic Stress Clinic, 1998), p. 5. Rumi, *The Essential Rumi*, translated by Coleman Barks (London: Penguin Books, 1995), p. 278.

PART III

Epigraph. "Katherine Anne Porter: Conversations," in *The Virago Book of Spirituality: Of Women and Angels*, ed. by Sarah Anderson (London: Virago Press, 1997), pp. 19-20. Virginia Woolf, *Moments of Being: A Collection of Autobiographical Writing*, ed. by Jeanne Schulkind (New York: Harcourt Brace, copyright © 1985, 1976 by Quentin Bell and Angelica Garnett), p. 69. Paramahansa Yogananda, *Autobiography of a Yogi* (Los Angeles, CA: Self-Realization Fellowship, 1946), p. 429. Thomas Merton, *No Man is an Island*, in *God in All Worlds: An Anthology of Contemporary Spiritual Writing*, ed. by Lucinda Vardey (New York: Pantheon, 1995), p. 551. Gary Zukav, *The Seat of the Soul* (New York: Fireside Books, 1990), p. 45. Dylan Thomas, *The Poems of Dylan Thomas* (NY: New Directions, 1971), p. 77. Hans Küng, "Once I have decided..." in *God in All Worlds: An Anthology of Contemporary Spiritual Writing*, ed. by Lucinda Vardey (New York: Pantheon, 1995), p. 14. "Meaningful coincidences..." source unknown, possibly *Was Carl Jung a Mystic?* Julian of Norwich, *Revelations of Divine Love* (London: Methuen & Company, 1901), p. ?

PART IV

Epigraph. T.S. Eliot, "Four Quartets, Little Gidding," *Collected Poems* 1909-1962 (London: Faber and Faber Ltd, 1963), p. 222. Nomadic principles, Jacques Attali, *The Labyrinth in Culture and Society* (Berkeley, CA: North Atlantic Books, 1999; Paris: Librairie Arthème Fayard, 1996), p. 77. Thomas Merton, in Nancy Louise Frey, *Pilgrim Stories: On and Off the Road to Santiago* (Berkeley: University of California Press, 1998), p. 79. Labyrinths: Watering Holes for the Spirit." Keynote address given by Reverend Dr. Lauren Artress, Glastonbury, 2002.

RESOURCES

BOOKS
Rape & Trauma
Maryanna Eckberg, *Victims of Cruelty: Somatic Psychotherapy in the Treatment of Post-traumatic Stress Disorder* (Berkeley, CA: North Atlantic Books, 2000)

Claudia Herbert and Ann Wetmore, *Overcoming Traumatic Stress: A Self-Help Guide Using Cognitive Behavioral Techniques* (New York: NYU Press, 2001)

Judith Herman, M.D., *Trauma and Recovery* (New York: Basic Books, 1997)

Linda E. Ledray, *Recovering from Rape* (New York: Henry Holt & Company, 1994)

Peter A. Levine, *Waking the Tiger: Healing Trauma* (Berkeley, CA: North Atlantic Books, 1997)

Aphrodite Matsakis, *I Can't Get Over It: A Handbook for Trauma Survivors* (Oakland, CA: New Harbinger Publications, 1996)

Aphrodite Matsakis, *Trust After Trauma: A Guide to Relationships for Survivors and Those Who Love Them* (Oakland, CA: New Harbinger Publications, 1998)

Babette Rothschild, *The Body Remembers: The Psychophysiology of Trauma and Trauma Treatment* (New York: W.W. Norton & Company, 2000)

Glenn R. Schiraldi, *Post-Traumatic Stress Disorder Sourcebook* (Los Angeles, CA: Lowell House, 2000)

Gloria Wade, *Hurting and Healing* (London: Chrysalis Books, 2001)

Robin Warshaw, *I Never Called it Rape: The Ms. Report on Recognizing, Fighting, and Surviving Date and Acquaintance Rape* (New York: Harper & Row, 1988)

Scriptotherapy

Louise DeSalvo, Ph.D., *Writing as a Way of Healing: How Telling Our Stories Transforms Our Lives* (San Francisco: HarperCollins, 1999)

Suzette Henke, *Shattered Subjects: Trauma and Testimony in Women's Life-Writing* (New York: St. Martin's, 1998)

James W. Pennebaker, *Opening Up: The Healing Power of Confiding in Others* (New York: William Morrow and Company, Inc., 1990)

Labyrinths

Reverend Dr. Lauren Artress, *Walking a Sacred Path: Rediscovering the Labyrinth as a Spiritual Tool* (New York: Riverhead Books, 1995)

Jacques Attali, *The Labyrinth in Culture and Society: Pathways to Wisdom* (Berkeley: North Atlantic Books, 1999; Paris: Librairie Arthème Fayard, 1996)

Helen Curry, *The Way of the Labyrinth: A Powerful Meditation for Everyday Life* (New York: Penguin Putnam, 2000)

Penelope Reed Doob, *The Idea of the Labyrinth: From Classical Antiquity Through the Middle Ages* (New York: Cornell University Press, 1993)

Reverend Dr. Jill Kimberly Hartwell Geoffrion, *Living the Labyrinth: 101 Paths to a Deeper Connection with the Sacred* (Cleveland, OH: The Pilgrim Press, 2000)

Hermann Kern, *Through the Labyrinth: Designs and Meanings Over Five Thousand Years* (New Jersey: Prestel Publishing, 2000)

Sig Lonegren, *Labyrinths: Ancient Myths and Modern Uses* (New York: Sterling Publishing Company, 2001)

W.H. Matthews, *Mazes and Labyrinths: Their History and Development* (New York: Dover Publications, 1985, reprinted from 1922 edition)

Helen Raphael Sands, *The Healing Labyrinth: Finding Your*

Path to Inner Peace (London: Gaia Books, 2001)

Jeff Saward, *Ancient Labyrinths of the World* (Thundersley, Essex, England: Labyrinthos, 1999)

Melissa Gayle West, *Exploring the Labyrinth: a Guide for Healing and Spiritual Growth* (New York: Broadway Books, 2000)

Labyrinth Journals

Caerdroia: The Journal of Mazes and Labyrinths, published by Labyrinthos, 53 Thundersley Grove, Thundersley, Benfleet, Essex, SS7 3EB, England

Labyrinth Web Sites

Caerdroia www.labyrinthos.net

The Labyrinth Society www.labyrinthsociety.org

Veriditas www.gracecathedral.org

Spirituality

Angeles Arrien, Ph.D., *The Four-Fold Way: Walking the Paths of the Warrior, Teacher, Healer, and Visionary.* (San Francisco: HarperSanFrancisco, 1993)

William Bloom, ed., *The Penguin Book of New Age and Holistic Writing* (London: Penguin Books, 2000)

Jean Shinoda Bolen, M.D., *The Millionth Circle: How to Change Ourselves and the World* (Berkeley, CA: Conari Press, 1999)

Pema Chödrön, *Start Where You Are* (Boston & London: Shambhala, 1994)

Phil Cousineau, *The Art of Pilgrimage* (Berkeley, CA: Conari Press, 1998)

Eckhart Tolle, *The Power of Now: A Guide to Spiritual Enlightenment* (London: Hodder & Stoughton, 2002)

ORGANIZATIONS
Dealing with Rape, Sexual Abuse, or PTSD

UNITED KINGDOM
of Great Britain & Northern Ireland

Mind (National Association for Mental Health)
Granta House
15-19 Broadway
London E15 4BQ
Phone: (0)20 8519 2122
E-mail: contact@mind.org.uk
Web: www.mind.org.uk
  ⁓*leading mental health charity which publishes "Understanding Post-traumatic Stress Disorder" and other useful leaflets*

The Oxford Stress and Trauma Center
8a Market Square
Witney, Oxon OX25 6BB
Phone: 01993 779007
Web: www.oxdev.co.uk
  ⁓*PTSD treatment for private patients*

Rape and Sexual Abuse Support Centre
P.O. Box 383
Croydon CR9 2AW
Helpline (0)20 8683 3300
Web: www.rasasc.org.uk
  ⁓*free, confidential and non-judgmental help and support for women and girls who have been raped or sexually abused, however long ago*

Rape Crisis Federation
Unit 7 Provident Works
Newdigate Street

Nottingham NG7 4FD
Phone: 0115 900 3560
E-mail: info@rapecrisis.co.uk
Web: www.rapecrisis.co.uk
～*multi-faceted referral service working to end rape*

Traumatic Stress Clinic
73 Charlotte Street
London W1T 4PL
Phone: (0)20 7530 3666
Web: www.traumaclinic.org.uk
～*PTSD treatment for NHS patients*

Women Against Rape
Crossroads Women's Centre
230a Kentish Town Road
London NW5 2AB
Phone: (0)20 7482 2496
～*activist organization offering support, counseling, legal advice, and information*

Women's Aid
P.O. Box 391
Bristol BS99 7WS
Phone: 0117 944 4411
Helpline: 08457 023 468
Web: www.womensaid.org.uk
～*national charity working to end violence against women and children*

The Women's Therapy Centre
10 Manor Gardens
London N7 6JS
Advice and Information Line: (0)20 7263 6200
E-mail: info@womenstherapycentre.co.uk
Web: www.womenstherapycentre.co.uk
～*provides therapy services by women for women, irrespective of race, cultural background, age, class, sexuality, income, or disability*

UNITED STATES

Department of Public Health
⁓*contact your local city, county, or state rape crisis/ treatment center and confidential counseling phone line*

The International Society for Trauma Stress Studies
60 Revere Drive, Suite 500
Northbrook, IL 60062
Phone: (847) 480-9028
Web: www.istss.org
⁓*professional network which shares knowledge of all aspects of the effects of trauma*

National Mental Health Association
1021 Prince Street
Alexandria, VA 22314
Phone: (703) 684-7722
Information Center: (800) 969-NMHA
Web: www.nmha.org
⁓*addresses all aspects of mental health and mental illness, including Post-traumatic Stress Disorder*

RAINN (Rape, Abuse, and Incest National Network)
635-B Pennsylvania Avenue, SE
Washington, D.C. 20003
Phone: (202) 544-1034
Hotline: (800) 656-HOPE
Web: www.rainn.org
E-Mail: rainnmail@aol.com
⁓*an excellent starting point, especially for those in crisis (including those in other countries), co-founded by singer/songwriter Tori Amos*

Rape 101
Web: www.rape101.com
⁓*an educational and enlightening web site*

Yellow Pages (phone book)
⁓*see the listings under "rape" for crisis intervention, counseling centers, women's organizations, etc.*

YWCA of the U.S.A.
Empire State Building
350 Fifth Avenue, Suite 301
New York, NY 10118
Phone: (212) 273-7800
Web: www.ywca.org
⁓*provides referrals to local programs and services for battered women and survivors of rape and sexual assault*

Acknowledgments

*Grateful acknowledgment is given to the
following for permission to use illustrations:*

front cover photo, Chalice Well Gardens, Glastonbury, courtesy of Regina Coppens-Koot.

page 10, copyright © 1969 by Roger Smith.

page 22, by Napoleon Sarony, courtesy of the Library of Congress, Prints and Photographs Division, LC-USZ62-73396.

page 74, by Sir John Everett Millais, copyright © Tate Gallery, London/Art Resource, NY.

page 93, copyright © 1989 by Quantity Postcards, Oakland, CA 94607.

page 109, from the author's private collection.

page 114 & back cover, courtesy of Veriditas: The Worldwide Labyrinth Project, Grace Cathedral.

page 146, source unknown.

page 153, by George Frederic Watts, copyright © Tate Gallery, London/Art Resource, NY.

page 191, adapted by Camille Flammarion from a 16th-century German woodcut.

page 207, floor mosaic, National Gallery, London, copyright © 2002 by Alice Whytefeather.

page 212, copyright © 2002 by Alice Whytefeather.

page 227, from Francis Quarles's 15th-century *Emblems*.

Pansies courtesy of a synchronistic meeting with a young Lithuanian woman in a London tearoom.

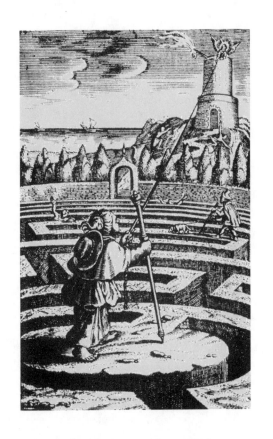

𝕭lessings on your path!

It begins with a story, untold.
It begins with a breath,
held for centuries
in one woman's heart.
It begins with silence
and ends, not with a scream,
but with one unfrozen tear of gratitude…

Alice Whytefeather is a spirit name. It came to me over time, during the writing of this book. I found that, by honoring my higher self imaginatively, I was freed to create and disclose in a way that was beyond the purely confessional. Alice is myself, yes, but she could be AnyWoman. I owe much to that great little shamanic adventurer, Alice in Wonderland, who descends through the rabbit-hole into chaos, only to rise up again. And, because of my appreciation of angels, I naturally gravitated to the surname Whytefeather, which symbolizes the charmed white feather of an angel's wing. Once, on the stone floor of Chartres Cathedral, I found such a specimen. Taking it in hand, I was reminded of a quill pen (though these were commonly fashioned from the flight feathers of geese, not angels). A medieval scribe working on an illuminated manuscript had to stop every few pages to trim her quill and thus sharpen the point; it must have demanded inkwells of patience. Perhaps writing has never been easy. Yet my only real task was to let myself be guided. May this book have wings.

www.risktoblossom.com